"Intuition is our birthright, and we can either ꜱᴏᴍᴇᴇ ᴇ choose to respect and develop this inner wisdom, our lives will be more joyful and fulfilled, and we can be of greater service to others. Francesca McCartney is a skillful guide in the task of refining this ancient way of knowing."

— Larry Dossey, MD,
author of *Reinventing Medicine* and *Healing Words*

"*Body of Health* skillfully lays out a practical path for cultivating your intuitive powers. Beyond the superb theory and methods, Francesca's personal story pulls you into your own intuitive depths. I recommend this book wholeheartedly."

— Donna Eden, author of *Energy Medicine*

"Dr. McCartney defines our bioenergetic nature and guides us to boldly explore what we intuitively know, yet only rarely dare admit. *Body of Health* acknowledges and embraces our entire self, going beyond philosophy and into the realm of lifestyle practice. It is more than an owner's manual for human beings that reminds us what we are and provides directions for our return to wholeness; it is also a recipe for cosmic healing."

— Len Saputo, MD, founder of Health Medicine Institute
and co-editor of *Boosting Immunity*

"Body of Health is chock-full of simple exercises to remind you that your intuitive skills are always present, patiently waiting for your attention. Francesca McCartney provides an excellent survey of practical techniques and lore about the connections between intuition and health."

— Dean Radin, PhD, senior scientist, Institute of Noetic
Sciences, and author of *The Conscious Universe*

"This book is a potent guide to opening up to the innate wisdom that we all possess. Body of Health is one of those rare books packed with the kind of usable information to help you lead a full, balanced, and creative life."

— Marcia Emery, PhD,
author of *PowerHunch* and *The Intuitive Healer*

BODY *of*
HEALTH

BODY *of* HEALTH

The New Science of INTUITION MEDICINE® for Energy & Balance

FRANCESCA McCARTNEY, PhD

FOREWORD BY C. NORMAN SHEALY, MD, PhD

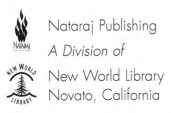

Nataraj Publishing
A Division of
New World Library
Novato, California

Nataraj Publishing

A Division of

New World Library
14 Pamaron Way
Novato, California 94949

Front cover design by Mary Ann Casler
Text design by Bill Mifsud
Mandala design by Peter Patrick Barreda (www.mandalazone.com)
Illustrations and charts by Christina Nelson

Library of Congress Cataloging-in-Publication Data
McCartney, Francesca.
  Body of health : the new science of intuition medicine for energy and balance / Francesca McCartney.—1st ed.
    p.   cm.
Includes bibliographical references and index.
ISBN 1-57731-488-3 (pbk. : alk. paper)
  1. Healing. 2. Intuition. 3. Vital force—Therapeutic use. 4. Self-care, Health. I. Title.
RZ999.M3658 2005
615.8'51—dc22   2005000993

First Printing, June 2005
ISBN 1-57731-488-3
ISBN-13 978-157731-488-2
Printed in the United States

New World Library is dedicated to preserving the earth and its resources. We are now printing 50% of our new titles on 100% chlorine-free postconsumer waste recycled paper. As members of the Green Press Initiative (www.recycledproducts.org/gpi/), our goal is to use 100% recycled paper for all of our titles by 2007.

10 9 8 7 6 5 4

To Zoe and Zena,
with love

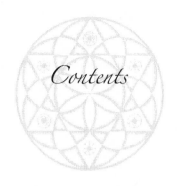

Contents

Foreword

by C. Norman Shealy, MD, PhD   xiii

Introduction

Intuition Medicine   1

Chapter 1

It Is in My Blood   11

Chapter 2

Indications of Intuitive Awareness   21

Chapter 3

Assessing Our Intuitive Abilities   31

Chapter 4

Intuition and Grounding: Grounding Is Good Medicine   39

Chapter 5

The Grounding Meditation Practice   61

Chapter 6

Meditation Sanctuary: Meditation Is a Location   71

Chapter 7

The Meditation Sanctuary Practice   99

Chapter 8

Life-Force and Earth Energy: Your Personal Healing Energy   105

Chapter 9

The Life-Force and Earth-Energy Meditation Practice   131

Chapter 10

The Chakra System: Physical and Spiritual Health   141

Chapter 11

The Chakra System Practice   167

Chapter 12

The Aura: Halo of Light   177

Chapter 13

The Aura Meditation and Healing Practice   201

Chapter 14

Color: The Language of Energy   211

Chapter 15

The Color Meditation and Healing Practice   237

Afterword   245

Appendix 1
Intuition Medicine Health Issues Reference Chart   249

Appendix 2
Chakra System Reference Charts   257

Acknowledgments   279

Endnotes   281

Bibliography   293

Index   301

About the Author   315

Foreword

BY C. NORMAN SHEALY, MD, PhD

*N*othing is more important to a fulfilling life than health, which is one of the greatest blessings we have. The facts are clear: at least 85 percent of all illnesses are the result of an unhealthy lifestyle. Drugs and surgery are occasionally helpful in treating illness; but maintaining health is your responsibility – and is a probability if you follow the program in *Body of Health*.

Listening to your intuitive intelligence provides the foundation for a healthy life. Dr. McCartney created the term Intuition Medicine and teaches how the best approach to remain healthy and to restore health is to develop your intuition to understand your body and its relation to mind, emotions, and spirit. *Body of Health* teaches you to be self-aware and healthy and to embrace intuition to transform your life.

Dr. McCartney's thorough explanation of the human energy system is exceptionally useful. From theory to integration, *Body of Health* provides useful tools for enhancing your personal intuitive healing. Building on a discussion of the wide variety of intuitive skills we all share, Dr. McCartney also provides useful self-assessment tools to evaluate your natural intuitive intelligence. Then you move into the critical practice of grounding or centering. You are introduced to physical, visual, and auditory methods that enhance intuition and meditative exercises. The rich variety of exercises provides a solid foundation for building your medicine chest of intuitive tools. The recommendation to keep an intuition journal is valuable in helping you develop your skills and provide you with feedback on your progress.

Body of Health is a marvelous antidote to the stress of modern life. With insights into energy blocks and clues to open them, here is your opportunity to study and practice the medicine of the twenty-first century — Intuition Medicine. Far more important than drugs, preventing illness and maintaining health are the keys to optimizing your life. I hope this brief overview of this gem of a book encourages you to read and practice the wisdom presented. Your health and happiness will be the happy recipients.

C. Norman Shealy, MD, PhD
President, Holos Institutes of Health, Inc.
President, Holos University Graduate Seminary
Founder, American Holistic Medical Association

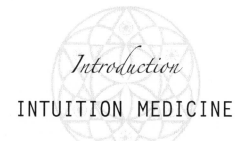

Introduction

INTUITION MEDICINE

Keeping your body healthy is an expression of gratitude to the whole cosmos — the trees, the clouds, everything.

— Thich Nhat Hanh

*H*uman beings are much more than bodies; our physical, emotional, and spiritual components are inextricably linked to create our personal universe. *Body of Health* presents a map for a human wholeness journey — a practice of living in health and balance, with all senses receiving gifts of guidance toward self-awareness while embracing the experience of the world. This, I believe, is what it means to live in a state of grace, and it calls for listening to your intuitive intelligence, your wisdom voice.

We live in a small world — an aggregated cosmology of reality, with personal universes entangled as one global consciousness. In this complex living organism, the health of one affects the whole. Many sciences and philosophies view the vital force of an individual as intrinsically linked with the collective whole, even given differences of time and distance. They see organisms as constantly exchanging energy and information with their surroundings in a complex field of life. At its best, this energetic interdependence brings strength when there are harmonious support systems and healthy communication. However, it can also be a cause of

1

dis-ease, especially for a sensitive individual when discord and destructive elements are present. *Body of Health* presents a whole-human perspective of wellness, grounded in the belief that health of the individual contributes to health of the whole.

Body of Health will teach you how to be self-aware and healthy in your body, mind, and spirit while living in a world abundant with diverse energies and people. By paying attention to the messages that you receive nonverbally through your body and through your own sensations, you can begin to appreciate your life on a deeper level. You will begin responding to your world in a new way, and the number and scope of the messages you receive will increase. This journey consists of listening to, trusting, and following your intuition. Your journey's guide, intuition, is the capacity to understand your interconnectedness in the universe with quick insight and direct knowledge.

INTUITIVE EXPLORATION

Becoming more aware of your intuitive sense changes your experience of life. This book is an invitation to participate in a transformative journey of intuitive exploration. When you embrace intuition along with your other five senses, your perspective on life opens up, you are presented with more possibilities, and you are given choices that directly influence your health, balance, and vital energy.

Read this book with the mind-set of an experimenter. Test the hypotheses, practice with new ideas, play with insights, and put what you learn into thought and practice. When you do this, your intuition will develop and work with your other senses. As your intuitive ability expands, you will tune into signals from each element of your being and discover how disturbances and changes in one area can affect your entire system.

In this book, I will introduce you to three essential methods for accessing your intuitive intelligence:

- Diagnosis or recognition: Owning your intuitive abilities and using them to diagnose your current state of health.

- Clearing and balancing: Increasing your level of overall health by clearing blockages and balancing your energy.

- Protection or self-possession: Creating a positively charged protection field in and around your personal universe and claiming full possession of your energetic space.

Like the elements of your personal universe, these categories cannot be neatly delineated; as you develop your skills in one area, your abilities in the other areas will improve and your entire intuitive awareness will be transformed.

With practice and observation, you will begin to see how energetic systems operate. In the same way that musicians increase the sensitivity of their ears through exercises and training, you will learn to increase your intuitive abilities by working with the wisdom tools presented in this book.

The system of Intuition Medicine is a study of human consciousness. This body of work is presented as an empirical methodology that harkens back to the time before a rationalistic/linear/dualistic worldview took precedence in scientific research. Before this Cartesian approach gained dominance, the scientist's subjective experience was naturally included as part of research data, rather than being regarded as interfering with the validity of the results.

I hope that, as you read this book, your understanding of what it means to be human will greatly expand. I invite you to discover that the science of human consciousness is not a technique or methodology, but a process that reveals itself when given attention.

HOW TO USE THIS BOOK

The tools you will find in *Body of Health* are meant to be used creatively to heal, enhance, and design your life. I present the information on many levels so that everyone from the beginner to the advanced student of life can glean something new. My intention is that you will receive a fulfilling amount of information whenever you approach this work. This also allows you to read the book more than once, gaining more insight each time. In this way, the book is designed to support your growth as you practice the Intuition Medicine tools and discover more about yourself.

While you are free to use *Body of Health* in any way that works for you, I believe that the following suggestions will help you get the most from this journey.

Keep an Intuition Journal

You will benefit from creating a personal book specifically to track your intuitive development and language. Use a lined, bound journal or ringed notebook, whichever you prefer. Journaling will allow you to keep track of your insights from the intuitive inquiry lists that are found through the book. You can record your answers to questions that accompany the meditations and make notes of the personal intuitive language that will develop. One of the main purposes of keeping a journal is to build trust in your intuition and observations.

Read from Front to Back

I recommend that you read the chapters in order, at least the first time through this book; your absorption of material in later chapters will be enhanced if you have read the earlier ones. Please read this book as a presentation of a new science that asks you to think nonlinearly and outside of the usual boxes.

Once you have read the entire book, feel free to review any of the chapters in any order.

Reflect on the Theoretical Chapters

This book is structured around two types of chapters: "theory with stories" chapters and "practice with integration" chapters. In each theoretical chapter, you will find an exploration of a specific concept and related theories, interlaced with real-life stories that demonstrate the humanness of the material.

All the stories and lists that describe various ways to experience states of intuitive awareness in the book are written by students and practitioners of Intuition Medicine; I have collected these stories from their journals, personal communications, and questionnaires completed during their formal study of Intuition Medicine.

These chapters also include reflective portions in which I ask you to stop for a moment and connect the concepts you have just read about with your personal experience. I have found that doing so helps integrate intuition with our other senses. This approach is designed to move you into simultaneously knowing, feeling, and thinking — the steps that will aid your alignment with the subtle sense of intuition. Intuition is a learned life skill that develops when you pay attention to it.

The "theory with stories" chapters also include lists that I have developed over many years of teaching with the help of my students and other practitioners. You can use these lists to understand the language of intuition in order to interpret subtle interactions with others and to get a clearer sense of why you feel comfortable or uncomfortable in various situations. Originally used, in part, to assess my methods and their effectiveness in helping others learn these skills, they eventually served as self-assessment tools for students. As you work with the exercises and techniques in the book, they can serve as a way to describe your own experiences with intuition. If these lists seem tedious the first time you read them, come back to them when they offer pertinent knowledge and healing. I trust that your intuition will direct you to revisit these lists when the information holds value for you.

Practice with the Integration Chapters

The "practice with integration" chapters include formal step-by-step meditations, questions to answer before and after meditation, daily awareness practices, experiments, and affirmations. The meditations are quite detailed; I do not expect you to sit with the book on your lap and meditate while reading each step (however, if that works for you, please do so!). I suggest that you read the steps of the meditation, then close the book and intuitively move through it by following what you recall; with repeated practice, you will create a personal contemplative ritual that works for you. If you prefer, you can record the meditations on an audiotape and play them back to guide your meditation. Or you may purchase my guided meditation audio recordings by visiting my website at www.intuitionmedicine.org.

You may want to set aside a regular meditation time on a daily or weekly basis to do the guided meditations, as if you were in a formal class. Or you may consider being flexible about the meditation practices, reading the book and doing the meditations when you feel the need or have the time.

Before you do the guided meditations, it is a good idea to prepare your space and yourself. Choose a comfortable location where you will not be disturbed. Draw the shades or dim the lights. Turn off the telephone. Put a "do not disturb" sign on your door. Then take a few moments to get into a calm, quiet mood. Put aside as many of your daily concerns as you can, and bring all your attention into the present moment and your present activity. Then, when you feel calm and quiet, begin the meditation. After completing the post-meditation questions and exercises, you may want to write any additional thoughts or comments in your journal. Your journal will become your personal book for the language of intuition.

In addition to doing the guided meditations, set aside a short, quiet meditation time each day. Just five to ten minutes daily will make a huge difference in your intuitive development. Some people meditate for a few minutes in the morning; others do it before going to bed. Some schedule five minutes of meditation into their lunch breaks. Intuit the best time and frequency for your personal meditation, and follow through on the answers you receive.

In each "practice" chapter, you will also find experiments, affirmations, and techniques. Play with the "Try This!" experiments as a "prove it to yourself" activity. Or you might want to spend an entire day simply repeating the affirmations from one of the practice chapters or focusing on one technique, such as grounding. The next day, focus on a different technique, such as communicating from your meditation sanctuary. At the end of the day, note the difference in your attitude, awareness, and general health.

Stay Aware Every Day

Each day, pay attention to your intuitive insights as they occur; many significant discoveries have been made during self-reflective moments, when the quick, clear "I know this!" intuitive insight occurs. Pay attention to the subtleties of life, as wisdom is a quiet invocation.

As with any new skill, practice is an important part of the learning process. You will find that Intuition Medicine will naturally become part of your daily life. Intuition Medicine is a body of health to be lived every day. But you can expedite that process by working with these tools on a daily basis. Focusing several times a day on any of the exercises will help you more quickly integrate this intuitive work into your life.

As you become more familiar with this body of health work, you will find yourself naturally stopping to meditate and using the skills throughout your day. You will take time to use the health tools before a big meeting, interview, or date. Or you will stop before visiting someone who tends to leave you unbalanced. Whenever you notice something amiss in your energy system, you will give yourself the time you need.

Trust Yourself

Remember that these are only guidelines. Everyone learns in different ways. If your intuition suggests an alternative, by all means trust yourself. Perhaps you need to read the entire book before doing the meditations. Or maybe you need to answer all the questions, read the book, and then go back and practice the exercises. There is no right or wrong way to do this. Trust your intuition.

AN OVERVIEW OF THIS BOOK

Body of Health begins with my personal story. This chapter describes how I first encountered my own perceptions of intuition and what it had to teach me. These experiences prompted me to begin my studies, and eventually led me to teaching and research. They are included as part of my vitae of teaching and writings.

In chapter 2, I explain the various types of intuitive awareness. Chapter 3 provides an easy and fun self-assessment tool that will give you a baseline against which to measure your aptitude for operating with your intuitive sense. I give the same test as part of the entrance requirement for the three-year Intuition Medicine program which I am the founder and president of. If some of the technical language in this chapter or any others, is uninteresting to you I encourage you to skip over it and move on to the rest of the chapters.

Subsequent chapters focus on aspects of the human energy system and its intuitive health. In my experience, caring for your energy anatomy is as vital to your health and well-being as caring for your physical anatomy. To help you acknowledge and work with your energy anatomy, I provide a series of information and practice chapters to acquaint you with the processes of Intuition Medicine. These chapters include charts and diagrams to assist you in visualizing what I am writing about. The charts will show you how I clairvoyantly see the energy anatomy systems.

In chapters 4 and 5, I explain how grounding is your emotional centering connection. Strong grounding will provide you with a stable foundation of well-being from which to operate in your daily life and contemplatively explore other components of your energy system.

Chapters 6 and 7 present the concept of meditation as a physical location in your body where you train yourself to rest your attention. This practice will allow you to function with a perception of living in the present moment.

Chapters 8 and 9 introduce my methodology of using life-force energy and earth energy as your personal healing energies. Life-force energy is your personal signature energy; it is unique to you, just like your fingerprint. The earth emits a natural electromagnetic energy, which has a healing effect on our bodies. The blend of these energies supplies you with vital force and emotional strength.

Chapters 10 and 11 acquaint you with chakras as the focal points of your energy system; imagine them as your personal computers of energy and information. The chakras act as input/output devices, determine how you communicate with others, and regulate your internal energy flow. Chakra balance is a major key to good health.

Chapters 12 and 13 discuss your aura — an energy skin and protection system that is filled with healing frequencies. This cocoon of vital light surrounding your body is like a woven energy garment, without which you are vulnerable to the energy of the world around you. The aura functions as protection, as an emotional boundary, and as a closed-circuit solar accumulator that maintains a healing energy resonance.

Chapters 14 and 15 end the book with an exposition of and practice in the use of color in meditation and healing. Color and light have long been recognized as powerful healing energies and tools for personal growth and healing. I give you practical information about how you can sense your moods as colors and shift your moods by changing your energy colors via intention and meditation.

The appendixes further deepen your knowledge about how your subtle energy system affects your health. The "Health Issues Reference Chart" offers direction on how to use the information in this book for specific health problems. I gathered the information in this chart from my energy work with thousands of people over the past thirty years. You can use the chart as a reference guide for your own exploration in healing.

The "Chakra System Reference Charts" are richly layered with life-enhancing information. These lists hold the sort of practical material that you can use every day, enabling you to function as a healthy person physically, mentally, emotionally, and spiritually.

I find that a serious student of any discipline will use a bibliography as a resource for further study. Thus, I include a bibliography detailing both the books I reference within this book and those that have influenced my work.

Body of Health is a compendium of wisdom-based knowledge on the art of living. Welcome, and good health to you.

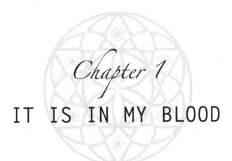

IT IS IN MY BLOOD

*I*ntuition flows in the blood of the women in my family. My paternal grandmother read the candle flame and people's minds. Stories of visitations from the spirits of dead relatives were passed around the dinner table between plates of pasta and eggplant. My mother read cookbooks and occult books. Her worn book on palmistry, *The Book of the Hand* by Fred Gettings, was passed on to me. Her advisors were card readers who used the red-and-black playing card deck. In my mother's last card reading, her advisor laid out seven cards on the table — every one of them was black. She died two weeks later. In that March card reading, she was told that a family wedding would occur in October; seven months later my father remarried. On the day my mother died, she telephoned our Catholic parish priest requesting that he call out her name on the prayer list so that the congregation would pray for her at morning Mass. My aunt attended that Mass and heard the priest ask the congregation to pray for her sister, who did in fact die late that night.

In old-world European tradition, "Catholic-occultism" was one term. I loved the rituals of Catholicism and devotedly followed all its precepts.

I was an extremely sensitive child, feeling, hearing, and seeing too much. The impact of my inner sensing system was so loud and distracting that I barely spoke for eighteen years. Of my fifty-one first cousins, I was the oldest girl and the quietest.

At nineteen, I had an epiphany during a Sunday Mass: I felt a deep awareness that the church prayers and sermons could no longer support my growing need to practice a religion of the spirit. I could no longer believe that only people baptized in the Catholic Church would go to heaven. A month later, a friend handed me the *Bhagavad Gita*, an East Indian book on spirituality. Never having been exposed to religious thought other than the Bible, I was surprised that I felt and understood the entire message of that book.

The cerebral stimulus of reading the *Bhagavad Gita* caused me to have a spontaneous energy opening. Heat rushed up my spine and out the top of my head in a rainbow — an explosion of fireworks. I found myself pushed out of my body, eyes wide open, in the middle of a starry sky, feeling "I am one with the universe." "Kundalini," an inner voice said. It was a new word for me, so I looked it up in the dictionary. To my surprise, it defined the word as a yogic life force that is held at the base of the spine until it is aroused and sent to the head to trigger enlightenment. I read more about kundalini in the *Bhagavad Gita*, and I realized that I had experienced a mystical awakening.

After my kundalini opening, I began to meditate naturally and frequently. When these mystical meditation experiences enraptured me, I knew how to go inside and listen, see, and feel, as that state had been my lifelong primary residence. In one spontaneous meditation episode, I asked, "What is my path in this lifetime?" A clear, feminine voice replied, "You are to heal people by reading the colors in their auras." I was twenty years old, it was 1967, and there were no classes offered at my university on aura reading. I did not know what the message meant. And so my healing apprenticeship began.

I did not start my search with the goal of becoming a healer, a medical intuitive, or an energy teacher. I was breaking through into a new personal investigation of consciousness, a rebirthing of myself led by listening to my hunches, my intuition. As a freshman at Wayne State

University in Detroit, Michigan, I entered the liberal arts program. The next year, I moved to Ann Arbor, Michigan, where I lived with some high school friends who were nursing students. I enrolled in a laboratory technician training program at the community college and specialized in hematology. Again, blood was guiding my way. During my internship training at St. Joseph Mercy Hospital, I became adept at intravenous needle insertion and drawing blood painlessly. I was always the technician chosen to draw blood from newborn babies. This field of study was stimulating, from preparing slides and using the microscope for blood-count analysis to assisting doctors during autopsies. I was literally seeing and investigating the inside of the human body.

That year, I met and married my first husband and we chose to move to a warmer climate. The University of California at Santa Barbara greeted us with a sunny change. I felt a strong desire to teach children, so I switched my major to preschool education and earned a Montessori teaching credential.

In Ann Arbor, a friend had introduced me to a meditation practice called Divine Science of the Soul, a Hindu mind-focusing practice. In Santa Barbara, I found a Divine Science teacher who held regular meditation meetings. During the formal initiation ritual, I heard church bells ringing loudly. Later I asked the teacher where the nearest church was, and he said there was none nearby.

I was fervent in my desire to discover the spiritual mysteries of Divine Science of the Soul. I rose early each morning and sat in lotus position for one hour, listening for the "sound current" and looking for the "inner light." The goal of this meditation was to move up to higher planes of spiritual enlightenment, as gauged by one's experience of seeing specific spiritual symbols, meeting deities, and hearing celestial sounds. My natural clairvoyance (the ability to see auras around bodies) and clairaudience (the ability to hear subtle sounds) magnified with this practice. This meditation practice began to refine my skill at traveling the inner pathways and circuits of my body, mind, and spirit.

My inner self was particularly interested in watching a thought or emotion emerge within my body and following its path from the origin of the feeling to its destination. I began to map the inner diagnostics of emotions, and a panoply of patterns, blueprints, and energy anatomies emerged. The teacher was not pleased with my veering off the focus of the meditation methodology.

In a personal audience, I received *darshan*, or blessing, from the master teacher of Divine Science of the Soul, Sant Kirpal Singh, when he visited the United States. I traveled with him and a group of devotees in a seven-month peace pilgrimage of meditation across the country. I later wrote to Sant Singh in Delhi for advice. His response was that clairvoyance and psychic abilities could be received only by the initiated gurus, and anyone else who pursued them was misusing power. I knew for certain that I was not a guru, and I was equally certain that I was not power-playing with what I felt to be a natural human ability.

I was practicing a science of the spirit and coming into a wealth of information on why I felt, thought, and responded in certain ways. Correlating what I had read about the focal energy points of the body, or chakras, with physical anatomy, an inner diagnostic blueprint began to evolve. At times, when I was sitting in deep contemplative meditation, an entire energy system with circuits and pathways would reveal itself to me, like a photographic film being developed in a darkroom. Intuitively, I began to intentionally heal sad memories by visualizing the energy circuit that had been imprinted with those memories, then dissolving them with currents of energy or affirmations. A feeling of loss often accompanied this dissolution, and I experimented with visualizing my highest healing currents restoring that area of my energy field to a better feeling — an upgraded electromagnetic energy-emotion.

I was so immersed in my inner life, rich with new discoveries, that I did not realize my marriage had self-destructed. I now had to choose between my wifely duties and my quest for spiritual engagement. I was selfish and chose to be alone. I moved to northern California and into a small cottage on a hilltop, in the middle of two thousand acres of redwood forest. Friends who owned this pristine property lived in the main house across the road. The nearest town, population two hundred, was two miles down a logging road. I drove ten miles to the next town to teach in a Montessori school. People described me as "weird," "lonely," or "that mystic on the hill." I felt free — happy to be a lone modern mystic on an inner-space exploration.

This was soon after my mother's suicide, and I was still processing her death. Crying was a big part of my mourning process, and I cried every day, all day, for nine months. It was a spiritual birthing time, a time of self-renewal. My tears would stop miraculously when I walked into my Montessori classroom, and begin again in a torrent as soon as I left the school grounds. I was led to a local Reichian-bioenergetic chiropractor who worked on my body and my energy for a year. He became a friend, a therapist, and an important person in my life. For the next decade, we synchronistically found each other repeatedly, through many changes in location and career.

My intuitive experiences continued to evolve. I had more pronounced kundalini activation and some spontaneous, out-of-my-control episodes in public places, which confirmed people's opinions that I was weird. One day, while attending a Tai Chi class, where we practiced the slow dancelike movements designed to support health, I began to feel the fire of kundalini rushing up my spine. When it got to my head, I fell to the ground, convulsed into a fetal position, and began to cry uncontrollably. Sad memories flashed through my mind and faded. I dragged myself to the corner of the room and continued to sob. Fifteen nonplussed people silently moved through their Tai Chi postures while a wild woman wailed on the floor. Everyone left the class quickly that day, and the teacher gently patted me on the head as he left.

Two days later, at the same posture in Tai Chi class, I again felt the burning rush up my spine. "Oh, no, not again!" I thought to myself. Again, I convulsed and fell to the floor, but this time a cacophony of laughter rippled out of my mouth. I dragged myself to the corner again and rolled around laughing. At the end of class, everyone left even more quickly than before. Later that week, I walked into a friend's health food store. He hugged me and said he had heard that I was having a difficult time learning my Tai Chi moves. My modern mystical experiences were being viewed as bizarre psychotic episodes rather than spiritual blessings!

In the weeks that followed, I began to have out-of-body experiences during which I would find my awareness dislocated from my body and feel like I was floating somewhere away from my physical self, at times traveling to places unknown. Strong currents of energy pulsed through my body, keeping me awake for days. My mother's spirit visited and clearly communicated that she needed me to heal her! What did that mean? She was a spirit without a body, and she was asking me to heal her? I instinctively stretched out my arms to embrace her.

My mother and I are kindred spirits, with a shared body experience. I was once cradled in her life-giving womb and nurtured by her blood. Now I became the spiritual womb in which she would gestate, waiting for me to find a way to birth her into a new life. In Catholic iconography, St. Theresa is depicted holding a bouquet of roses, with an illuminated, pierced heart thrust forward. My mother's name was Theresa, she had a passion for growing roses, and she died of a broken heart — incapacitated by emotional sorrow.

The events that had brought me to that time in my Tai Chi class and to all that followed had been tragic and difficult. They had begun a year before, when I had flown home from my hilltop nest in northern California to Harper Woods, Michigan, looking forward to spending time with my family. December is icy-cold in Michigan, and my childhood home felt even colder inside. My father, Frank, had recently asked for a divorce, and my mother, Theresa, was devastated and deeply depressed. Chemical depression runs in the genes of our family, but at that time no research had been done on the biochemical nature of depression, and her doctor was simply prescribing sleeping pills. It was New Year's Eve at the countdown to midnight. My father was not at home that night, and my mother and I watched Guy Lombardo on the television, pointing to the glowing New Year's ball hanging above Times Square as people reveled in the streets. Sitting close to my mother on the sofa, I could hear the rhythm of her slow breathing. Earlier that night, we had talked about the pain of my own divorce and the healing that had followed. She did not feel that she could start a new life after a divorce; all she knew how to be was a mother and wife. Indeed, she had been a mother since age sixteen, obliged to raise her eight younger siblings when her own mother, Francesca, died of breast cancer. When Theresa married Frank at age twenty-seven, all of her siblings but one had married. She left her parents' home and brought her youngest sister into her new home, where I was born the next year.

The Times Square ball dropped. It was midnight, and I found myself inside my head, feeling enveloped by clairvoyant images. In this vision, I saw my mother swallowing a bottle of prescribed sleeping pills that she had been hoarding for months; now she was taking her last breath. I jumped out of that vision and grabbed Theresa, who had slumped over on the sofa. I shook her and yelled, "Wake up!"

She opened her eyes and looked at me.

"Mom," I said, "did you take sleeping pills tonight?"

"No, no, I'm just very tired," she said.

"Please," I begged, "promise me that you will not do anything to hurt yourself."

My mother and I were empathically connected that night. Months later, I would wonder with remorse if I might have emotionally transferred the idea of suicide to her. After my mother went to bed, I lay sobbing in a fetal position on the floor by her closed bedroom door. Frank arrived home at 3:00 AM. I told him of my feelings and my vision. His reply was "Why are you trying to make me feel guilty?"

Boarding the plane for California the next day, I looked in my mother's eyes and said, "I love you." I hugged my younger brother and asked him to promise to take care of our mother. Three months later, two days before her fifty-sixth birthday, my mother fulfilled my prophetic vision by taking her own life. We buried her on her birthday.

Frank was a big-band musician; six months after my mother's death, he married a blonde groupie — in October, as the card reader had predicted. After his remarriage, our family divided, and I found myself divorced from my father's new home.

A few months after my mother had died, I was asleep in my bed in northern California when I heard my mother call out, "Fran!" I was jolted from my sleep. *I heard my mother's voice calling my name!* I reached out instinctively to hug her. This was not telepathy; this was clairaudience. An energy image of my mother stood beside my bed. Our communication had always been good when she was alive, and now she had found a way to continue our relationship. From that point until now, I have received communications from my mother telepathically and in my dreams. But that night *I heard her voice audibly.* She appeared sad, tired, and in pain. She was asking me to help her. I felt on a deep level that I knew how to help her. And at that moment, in the middle of the night, with her voice still reverberating in my ears, all I could do was open my heart and embrace her.

My unfolding journey led me to study many modalities of spirituality, healing, and energy. I learned about the chakra system from a clairvoyant chiropractor who was a student of the East Indian mystic J. Krishnamurti. I studied the psychic alchemy of the teachings of the Rosicrucian Order from two imperators (high officials akin to bishops or rabbis), one of whom gave me his Rosicrucian monographs that held the secret rituals of this order. I apprenticed with practitioners of iridology, herbology, and Bach flower remedies. My desire to counsel dying patients in hospitals led to nonsectarian seminary training and my 1975 ordination as a pastoral minister. Within this seminary community, I connected with many healers practicing alternative medicine.

In 1976, I introduced the speakers at a conference entitled "Alternative Healing in the Bay Area." There I met neurologist Alan Charles, MD, who was a Zazen meditation practitioner and the physician for the Mt. Shasta Abbey monks. After becoming acquainted with my work, he invited me to join his alternative medicine clinic, the Academy of Eastern Medicine, in Walnut Creek, California. There, for the next seven years, I practiced as both meditation instructor and medical intuitive — the latter is a term that describes a health practitioner who combines intuitive insight with medical information or one who includes a spiritual perspective on physical illness. I use the words *spiritual* and *intuitive* interchangeably, with both referring to the subtle energy of a person rather than to biological or emotional energy. Through this work, I became one of the first professional intuitives to practice an interdisciplinary modality that combined Eastern and Western healing arts in a medical clinic. During my years at Dr. Charles's clinic, I studied numerous systems of alternative and complementary medicine such as radionics, ayurvedic medicine, homeopathy, and acupuncture. While studying acupuncture, I realized that my clairvoyant scans of human energy anatomy looked quite similar to the pattern of Chinese acupuncture meridians. In fact, one energy system I observed, which I named the Spiritual Incarnation System™, was exactly the same as the golden-needle Chinese medicine meridian called Receive Spirit.

In 1980, Dr. Charles and I gave a talk entitled "The Effects of Energy and Color in Health and Behavior" at the International Academy of Preventive Medicine's annual conference in Denver, Colorado. In it, we presented our clinical work on the efficacy of combining meditation, the chakra system, and color as a healing modality. In the clinic, Alan and I had combined our healing approaches to create a noninvasive modality for the patients he diagnosed with high blood pressure or stress-related illness.

I continued to work at the Academy of Eastern Medicine as well as privately with clients and taught at various schools of healing and psychic studies in California. In 1984, I resigned from the clinic and founded the Academy of Intuition Medicine. In 2002, I earned a dual doctorate degree in Energy Medicine and Intuition Medicine from Greenwich University.

My passion is teaching. Over the next decade, I taught thousands of students the system of Intuition Medicine — my synthesis of years of work and study in Eastern and Western spiritual and healing arts.

Maybe my body is wired differently than most. Everyone processes information and experiences life in his or her own way, and I have great respect for the uniqueness of each individual. At the same time, I have found many people who understand my energy language and my approach to healing and spirituality. I do not feel crazy or at cross-purposes with the reigning cultural paradigm. I trust my inner voice, and I walk through life with ease and grace. I am pushed by questions and a sense of purpose. I am compelled to dissect and examine human consciousness and to map my findings and experiential research along with other soul scientists. As I follow my journey, life surges with wisdom, insight, and the continuity of past, present, and future. My spirit and blood flow in a matrilineal path: my daughters have inherited and carry on my gifts of intuition and healing.

Chapter 2

INDICATIONS OF INTUITIVE AWARENESS

The intuitive mind is a sacred gift, and the rational mind is a faithful servant. We have created a society that honors the servant and has forgotten the gift.

— Albert Einstein

You possess intuitive intelligence — your "wisdom guide." Your intuitive intelligence is a pharmacopoeia of inner knowledge, a vital system infused with life and designed to create a state of health and well-being. You already know how to feel good about yourself; your wisdom intuitively guides you to seek harmony. Maybe you have forgotten how to find or use your wisdom language, but nevertheless it remains within you. Intuition is located in the inner universe of human perception. It is the language of this inner wisdom — the natural human sense of knowing. The dictionary defines *intuition* as "the faculty of knowing as if by instinct, without conscious reasoning."[1] Intuition is a sense of knowing without knowing how you know. Intuition is the "aha" you sometimes experience after racking your brain for a solution. Intuition is the light-bulb over your head. Intuition is the flash of insight that reveals where your misplaced keys are hidden. Intuition is seeing an image of your long-lost friend's face in your mind just before you meet on the street. Intuition is the small, quiet voice so often drowned out by the more insistent noises inside and out. It is the voice that advises us — the voice of which we often later say, "If only I had listened..." Intuition is a human sense that provides you with a heightened sensitivity to the world around you. This "sixth sense" works compatibly with the other five senses and provides you with an additional means of perception. All of us have the ability to be intuitive, though it is naturally more acute in some people.

INTUITION AND HEALING

Intuition has played a critical role in the evolution of humanity. Early societies would undoubtedly have perished without the ability to tap into the power of intuition. In the course of human evolution, people relied on instinct before they had language. Instinct preceded language. Visualization of images preceded formal thought, art, and language. We humans generally tend to process things instinctually before we process them verbally.

Many cultures discovered information about the world around them through quiet contemplation. They also gave places of honor to shamans, priests, and oracles, who relied on contemplative reverie as a means of seeking wisdom. Today indigenous cultures throughout the world still use various forms of intuition for healing and problem solving. And it is well documented that many great minds of science and medicine have received revolutionary insights through unreasoned, intuitive processes; only later were such insights proven valid in the laboratory. Today many alternative healing practitioners include their intuitive insights in the diagnostic profile of patients, and alternative healing programs include courses on intuition and indigenous healing as part of the curriculum.

Contemporary people who seek alternative paths to health are validating ancient practices and seeking information from books, teachers from ancient cultures, and indigenous healing practices. Our culture is now infused with a broad selection of alternative, holistic, and complementary care choices for health and healing based on ancient medicine.

The practice we now call traditional medicine is a comparatively new development in human history. However, in the past hundred years or so, it has been supported by a massive campaign for credibility, leaving little room for other healing arts. Chinese medicine, homeopathy, ayurvedic medicine, chiropractic, and other forms of "alternative medicine," which have been part of human history for centuries, have only recently become acceptable forms of treatment in our society. In the past decade, research funded by national institutions like the National Institute of Complementary and Alternative Medicine, which is a branch of the National Institutes of Health, and privately funded organizations like the Fetzer and Samueli Institutes supplies us with compelling statistics on the efficacy of these ancient practices in treating disease and promoting health and well-being.

While by no means a common practice, medical intuition is now being brought into hospitals, healing clinics, and medical offices. At California Pacific Medical Center in San Francisco, there is a medical intuitive on the staff of the Institute for Health and Healing. If a patient requests this type of healing support, the medical intuitive will sit inside or just outside the surgery room, maintain intuitive communication with the patient during treatment, and pray for or spiritually heal the patient. General practitioners are beginning to call on professional intuitives for advice or second opinions. In California, medical intuitives work at several integrative medicine clinics, such as the Health Medicine Institute in Lafayette, 9 Corners Center for Balanced Living in Novato, and Hill Park Clinic in Petaluma. A medical intuitive is also part of the innovative, spa-like dental office in Berkeley called Transcendentist. In Boston, Massachusetts, Ann McCluskey, a medical intuitive who is also a Registered Nurse, reports that she offers spiritual healing to her patients; in many cases, they respond so well that medication is cut back or eliminated.[2]

On its own, Intuition Medicine has alleviated many conditions for which traditional medicine had no diagnosis and has cured many illnesses that were considered untreatable. A few graduate educational institutions provide degrees and certification in medical intuition, offering academic, experiential, and research-based training.

TYPES OF INTUITION

How do you experience intuition? Are you aware when your sixth sense is at work? Do you take it for granted? Does it take you by surprise? Take a moment to consider how you experience your intuitive nature. Then look at the following list. This list provides a brief introduction to some of the ways in which you may experience intuition; it is by no means exhaustive. You may sense these modes of awareness in relation to yourself, to others, or to the world around you.

Clairvoyance: Clear Seeing

Clairvoyance is a "visual" experience or awareness of subtle energy. Common visual experiences may include colors, symbols, patterns, or images. With clairvoyance, you experience an awareness of energetic patterns. Often people see a halo of color or energy around a person's head; this is an experience of clairvoyance.

Clairaudience: Clear Hearing

Clairaudience involves hearing words, sounds, songs, or tones that are not within the range of normal hearing. This perception is experienced as an outer sound, as opposed to an inner mental thought. Clairaudience is also described as a human sonar system that allows you to hear unspoken sounds. Do you sometimes hear a person's voice — familiar or unfamiliar — as though someone were speaking to you, yet no one is there? If so, you may be clairaudient.

Clairsentience: Clear Feeling

Clairsentience is an acutely developed sense of empathy. This skill utilizes the nervous system to feel energy. Clairsentience is also referred to as body radar. If you are conversing with someone who is depressed and you begin to feel depressed or sad, or if you are feeling pain in your heart and then learn that your best friend just had a heart attack, you are experiencing clairsentience.

Telepathy: Mental Communication

Telepathy is communication without verbal/auditory speaking. This skill involves both sending and receiving. Perhaps you are driving home from work and you suddenly feel like picking up some ice cream for dessert. When you arrive home, your partner says that she was thinking about serving ice cream for dessert but found none in the refrigerator. You have received her telepathic thought.

Knowing: Abstract Sensing

Intuitive knowing presents answers and information, often in no logical manner. Knowing may be experienced as a certain feeling, awareness, or trust-based perception. You have the information, but you cannot explain in any logical manner how you received it. This is an intuitive process that comes as a certain feeling or awareness that you trust. It may be the "aha" that comes out of nowhere. Or it may be that crystal-clear awareness of the best course of action — a course that may make little or no logical sense.

Precognition: Future Perception

Precognition means the perception of future events. Precognitive information can be perceived by means of knowing, clairaudience, clairvoyance, telepathy, dreams, visions, or clairsentience. Precognition includes forecasting the future, be it the next minute, hour, day, or so on. If you dream of an old friend and then meet him on the street the following day, you have experienced dream precognition. If you follow a gut feeling to not go on a cruise, then find out that the boat sank, you have experienced a combination of clairsentience and precognition. Do you often say to yourself, "I knew that was going to happen"? If so, you are precognitive.

Psychometry: Contact Perception

Psychometry means the use of one's hands to sense energy. It is a form of dowsing — which uses implements like a willow rod held in the hands to locate water or a pendulum suspended over an object to meas-ure its energy — but psychometry does not require any attending objects. Therapeutic Touch, which is an alternative healing practice taught in most nursing schools, uses psychometry as a measurement instrument of health. Nurses are taught to move their hands about six inches away from the patient's body in order to scan weak and strong vibrational pulses of health.

INTUITION AS A WISDOM TOOL

Knowledge has three degrees: opinion, science, and illumination. The

means or instruments of the first is sense; of the second, dialectic; of the

third, intuition. This last is absolute knowledge founded on the identity

of the mind with the object known.[3]

— Plotinus

There are no distinct dividing lines among the various forms of intu-ition. If you know who is calling before the phone rings, it might be pre-cognition at work, or telepathy, or a knowing sense, or a bit of all three. You may experience some of these on a regular basis, and others rarely or never. And as you develop your intuition, some of these abilities that are now dormant will become active wisdom tools in your Intuition Medi-cine toolbox.

No matter which intuitive tools you use, it is important to recognize and honor your unique mode of intuitive awareness. Become conscious of the modes you utilize most often, as well as the ones that seem to be beyond your current abilities. Keep track of which situations trigger var-ious intuitive abilities within you.

Try to become aware of your use of intuition in your daily life. Con-gratulate yourself each time you open to your inner awareness.

SCIENCE AND BIOELECTRIC FIELDS

The new vision of reality comes very close to the views of mystics of all ages and traditions. In particular the views of the ancient wisdom of the East provide the most consistent philosophical background to our modern scientific theories.[4]

— Fritjof Capra

Every human generates a personal energetic field. Like radio antennae, we send and receive electromagnetic signals to and from the world around us. Spiritual systems and healing practices have long recognized the presence of this energy and have worked with it to promote well-being and healing. Modern science is catching up with these ancient practices by inventing machines that measure and direct bioelectric fields. The Kirlian camera, which photographs subtle energy fields, has been in use since the 1960s. The biofeedback machine, which was developed at the Menninger Clinic in the 1950s, measures brain-wave activity in response to stress-reduction therapy. A recent study published in *New Scientist* magazine found that the body's natural electricity can be amplified via an optical device implanted in the cornea of the eye, promoting faster healing.[5] Other subtle energy measurement devices invented in the past century include the voll meter (a radionics machine), the psychotechnics meter, resonant field imaging, and random number generators (used in research to measure subtle field changes, globally as well as in small spaces).

Paradigm-shifting research on the use of intuition in distant and non-local communication and the effect that humans can have on machines has been conducted since the 1970s at the laboratory of Princeton Engineering Anomalies Research. Other nonprofit organizations devoted to research and study in the fields of intuition, consciousness, and expanded human capabilities include the Society for Scientific Exploration, the Institute of Noetic Sciences, and the International Society for the Study of Subtle Energies and Energy Medicine.

ENVIRONMENTAL FACTORS

Imagine that your environment helps you to feel in touch with yourself,
peaceful, and connected with the pulse of life.[6]

— Carol Venolia

Sensitive people are tuned into the electromagnetic frequencies of other humans. Unfortunately, they are also tuned into other energy fields in their environment. Power lines, computers, radios, televisions, microwave ovens, and cellular telephones all fill the air with disruptive currents. In addition to the energy transmitted by these devices, which most of us live with, many people must deal with the disruptive energy of marginally functional relationships. Families, jobs, schools, and romantic partnerships can all introduce negative energy into our personal universe. All of these factors can cause sensitive people to feel overwhelmed and lose their natural sense of well-being.

Using Intuition Medicine, you can learn to recognize the effects of these external energy sources. As you become more aware of them, you will also discover how to provide a protective energy field for yourself, bring your sensitivity into balance, and create a personal state of health that remains constant no matter what the state of the world outside you might be.

THE INTUITIVE SENSE

We are not human beings on a spiritual journey. We are spiritual beings on
a human journey.[7]

— Stephen Covey

Your senses serve your health and healing. The more fully you operate, sense-alive in sight, smell, hearing, taste, touch, and intuition, the healthy and happier you will be. Many people ignore or simply do not pay attention to the intuitive sense. With the will to learn and the right coaching, you can develop your dormant intuitive sense. This book will assist you in that endeavor through a system that has been practiced successfully by thousands of people for the past twenty years.

As you embark on this inner journey, try not to have expectations. Accept the fact that your intuition will develop at the pace that is perfect for you.

Chapter 3

ASSESSING OUR INTUITIVE ABILITIES

We dream of traveling through the universe — but is not the universe
within ourselves? The depths of our spirit are unknown to us —
the mysterious way leads inwards. Eternity with its worlds — the past
and future — is in ourselves or nowhere.

— Novalis

You are already intuitive. Intuition is your birthright, along with your other human senses. No doubt you have had some of your other five senses "tested" for operational health. It is always fun and interesting to chart your sense-abilities, so I have created an easy test of your intuitive sense.

The following self-assessment tool will help you rate your intuitive skills and discover which ones you have developed more highly. As you practice Intuition Medicine, your dormant skills will develop and the ones you already use will become more refined.

I suggest that you complete this self-assessment before reading farther; it will create a benchmark for where you are now. Record your responses in your intuition journal (see the Introduction). As you develop your intuition, take the test again, as this will allow you to look back periodically to see how much progress you have made. Included in this chapter is a key to help you interpret the present state of your intuitive skills. Do not read this key before you do the self-assessment test if you want to receive accurate, objective information about your level of intuitive development.

31

SELF-ASSESSMENT TOOL

Mark your responses to the following statements on a scale of one to ten; one indicates that the statement is not true, and ten means that it is always true.

NOT TRUE   **OFTEN TRUE**   **ALWAYS TRUE**

o   I   2   3   4   5   6   7   8   9   IO

1. I use my intuition on a daily basis.

2. I listen to my quiet inner voice.

3. I trust my knowing sense.

4. I apply my intuitive awareness to all areas of my life.

5. I sense when I am grounded and centered in my personal space.

6. I know and sense the signature of my own personal energy.

7. I sense other people's energy in my personal space.

8. I sense the energy lingering/held in physical places.

9. I recognize the times and activities that diminish my energy integrity.

10. I know my spiritual truth.

11. I feel energies in my hands.

12. I feel energies in my body.

13. I see people's auras, patterns, light, and energy.

14. I cry when I listen to certain types of music.

15. I feel what others are feeling.

16. I sense mental images that hold information.

17. I sense mental messages from others.

18. I predict future situations.

19. I notice when synchronicity occurs in my life.

20. I trust and act upon my intuition.

21. I am receptive to Universal gifts.

22. I trust my visions.

23. When I touch an object, I receive information about it.

24. I can tell who is on the phone before I pick up the receiver.

25. My dreams often come true.

26. I hear sounds that are not within the range of normal hearing.

KEY TO THE SELF-ASSESSMENT TOOL

Use the following key to generally understand which of your intuitive skills are best developed or most often used, and which are your quieter, less-used intuitive skills. With practice and attention, you can develop all of them. Tally your results and use this scale to assess the current state of your intuitive skills: 0–1, undeveloped skill; 2–4, moderate development of skill; 5–7, good development of skill; 8–10, highly developed skill.

In the categories indicated below, several of the twenty-six statements can be related to more than one intuitive skill:

Clairaudience: 14, 26

Clairsentience: 5, 6, 7, 8, 12, 14, 15, 23

Clairvoyance: 9, 13, 16, 17, 22

Knowing: 1, 2, 3, 4, 5, 6, 7, 9, 10, 19, 20, 21

Precognition: 18, 20, 22, 25

Psychometry: 6, 7, 11, 12, 23

Telepathy: 14, 16, 17, 24

RESEARCH: AN ANALYSIS OF INTUITIVE SKILLS

In 2002, as my doctoral research, I conducted a study on the use of intuitive skills, later presented in several forums as "An Empirical Study of the Transmission of Healing Energy via E-mail."[1] The inspiration for this research came from an experience I had as a teacher of professional intuitives at the Academy of Intuition Medicine. The program provides each student with an alumnus mentor who assists in coursework and also gives weekly energy-systems healings to a student. An alumna of the 1993 program and a professor in the computer arts college of a German university worked with a student who was an owner of a computer consulting company.

The student had many areas of intuitive interest that matched well with the alumna's expertise. Given that they both spent a good deal of time at their computers and on the Internet, I decided to have them connect at a distance via email as student and mentor. I assumed that they would communicate via some live chat system, forgetting that the time difference between Germany and the United States would not allow for this kind of communication. They began, quite organically, to communicate to each other via text email as though they were speaking to each other in the present moment. The student would ask for an energy healing with specific requests regarding energy systems, and then send the email to the mentor. The mentor would receive the message — usually eight hours later — and respond by sending both a reply email text message and, encapsulated within that text, an energy healing. They were inspired to discover that the sending and receiving of energy-systems healings were operating as intended — without physical proximity.

For the sake of brevity and to keep to the topic of this book, I will address only the part of my doctoral research that most pertains to our discussion of intuitive awareness. As part of my research, I administered a test once a week, for four consecutive weeks, to eighty-eight professional intuitives, alumni of the Academy of Intuition Medicine, who were receiving a healing energy over a distance. The test involved detecting three different specific energies — a body, a mind, and a spirit healing energy, all of which are taught as part of the Academy training program. A fourth, "sham healing," with no energy, was incorporated into this test as a neutral control. This test was not sent to sick people seeking healing, but to trained intuitives familiar with these specific energies, as a test of the reception and identification of healing energy utilizing intuitive skills. All the energies were randomly sent from the Institute of Noetic Sciences laboratory by the Academy's graduate program instructor. The intuitives did not know who was sending the energy, where the sender was located, or on which day of each of the four weeks the energy would be sent. At least one alumnus from each of the Academy classes, from the first in 1986 to the most recent 2002 program, was part of the research; and they were located throughout the United States, Australia, and Ireland.

I was testing the ability of a person to, first, detect reception of distant healing energy and, second, qualify the specific type of healing energy received. If the test subjects detected the presence of a healing energy, the questionnaire that they were given as part of the test instructed them to identify the energy and then place checkmarks next to all the intuitive skills they had used in detecting the identified energy. Through this research, I found that people often use more than one intuitive skill at a time to enhance perception. The subjects were given this alphabetical list of seven intuitive skills to choose from:

1. Clairaudience

2. Clairsentience

3. Clairvoyance

4. Knowing

5. Precognition

6. Psychometry (detecting energy through the hands only)

7. Telepathy

Intuitive Skills Usage

The test results revealed that most subjects used different skills or combinations of skills each week. The four predominant skills used were knowing, clairsentience, psychometry, and clairvoyance. The other three skills — precognition, clairaudience, and telepathy — were used infrequently.

Two of the listed skills, clairaudience and telepathy, were never used alone by any of the test subjects; when they were used, it was always in combination with other skills. The other five skills were used both alone and in combination with other skills.[2]

Accuracy of Intuitive Skills

Are some intuitive skills more accurate than others? My research results showed that accuracy did not depend on the specific intuitive skill used.

I analyzed the results to determine whether the success rates were dependent on the intuitive skills that were used. The statistical results were highly insignificant, indicating that there is no supporting evidence that accuracy is dependent on the specific intuitive skill used. This leads me to assume that any intuitive skill or combination of skills can function with comparable accuracy.[3] Given this, I would say that whatever intuitive skills you have developed will most likely operate with a fair to good rate of accuracy.

YOUR INTUITIVE INTELLIGENCE QUOTIENT

Intuition is your acumen in perceiving the subtleties of the world. If you found that you scored high in your knowing sense on the self-assessment test, then you are using the intuitive skill that people use most. This *quick insight* will serve you well as a decision-making tool. The results of my research also confirm that clairsentience is a widely used and highly developed intuitive sense for many people. If you scored high on that skill, you are among a large group of people who intuitively feel the world.

I observe that most sensitive people pick up subtle information in their hands and yet are not aware of this psychometry ability, as my research showed psychometry rated third in usage. Most often, you combine two or more intuitive skills in harmony, as you no doubt already do with sight, smell, taste, touch, and hearing.

The information in this chapter is meant to show that intuitive skills can be tested and measured, and that with practice your body can be calibrated as a measurement instrument to determine your intuitive development. Intuition is a subtle energy sense and one that provides you with a new perspective on yourself and a wider range of awareness of the world.

Physicists, mathematicians, and physicians now perceive what artists and mystics have always known: human beings are made of energy. Thoughts, emotions, colors, disease, beauty, and spirituality all exist as energy. When we learn to manage the energy we are made of, we can heal in body, mind, and spirit. You are about to embark on a wonderful journey of self-discovery and well-being. This book offers you a new way to see yourself, your world, and your place within the universe. Take a moment now to congratulate yourself for your decision to deeply explore personal healing and intuitive intelligence. As you work with this information, remember to stop from time to time and notice all the positive changes you are making in your life. Honor yourself for the work you are doing. Trust that you are always doing what is best for you. Play with your imagination, intuition, and wisdom. And, most of all, have fun.

Chapter 4

INTUITION AND GROUNDING:
GROUNDING IS GOOD MEDICINE

The whole body aligns with gravity, feeling the head as if suspended from the stars above.

— Mantak Chia

*G*rounding benefits people of all ages and lifestyles. It is a free, natural inducer of emotional and physical health. Grounding helps you settle into yourself and create a calm mood when you are overwhelmed by people, activity, or your surroundings. Before you enter a potentially stressful situation, close your eyes, take a deep breath, and visualize your body as a redwood tree rooting you into the earth. Continue to imagine the roots settling you into the earth until you feel relaxed and your mind begins to clear. Use grounding to feel at home within yourself wherever you are.

The intuitive practice of grounding is a connection with the earth that provides health benefits, as it adds electrons to the human body and electrons are antioxidants.[1] Sensitive people benefit emotionally from the practice of grounding, especially if they tend to avoid social situations, feel overwhelmed by crowds and noise, feel uncomfortable leaving the house, or have difficulty focusing on grocery shopping.

Grounding is a simple practice, and it is easy to add to your meditation as an affirmation, visualization, sensation, or emotion. Once grounding is set into your system, it becomes a natural part of who you are and how you feel. In fact, you feel unnatural and uncomfortable when you are not grounded.

The Intuition Medicine practice includes connecting to the earth through four grounding anchor points: meditation sanctuary, the first chakra, the feet chakras, and the aura (see the Grounding Anchor Points illustration on the following page). The meditation sanctuary is where your spirit grounds within your body to fully experience life. The first chakra anchors your emotional energy into the earth, giving you a sense of calm and balance. The feet chakras are your connecting points to the physical world that strengthen your healing relationship with the earth. Grounding your aura into the earth creates a protective energy field between you and the world. A more thorough exposition on each of these grounding anchor points will be presented throughout the book.

Experiment with different images to ground yourself; change them daily or for different situations until you find the right fit for the day or the occasion. In emotional communications, you may feel the need for more fluidity; a waterfall image surrounding your body and holding you in an aura of protection could be helpful in such a case. In stressful or challenging situations, you might use a big, strong, braided metal cable of gold, silver, and copper anchoring your feet into the earth.

You can use some simple self-observations to know and feel whether you are grounded. If you feel frazzled and not quite focused on a task at hand, or if you turn from a graceful swan into a bit of a clod, these are clues that you may be ungrounded. In the kitchen, if you spill something, drop something, or forget to close a cabinet door and bump your head, there is a good chance that you are ungrounded. Forgetfulness is a clue as well, as when you cannot find keys, books, or phone numbers or you know that your timing is off. If you are not grounded when driving, you may miss an exit or your reflexes may not be quick when making a turn or parking. If you feel unsure of yourself, not centered, apprehensive, and shy when meeting people, these are clues that grounding is needed and will certainly help with your self-confidence. There is a dramatic

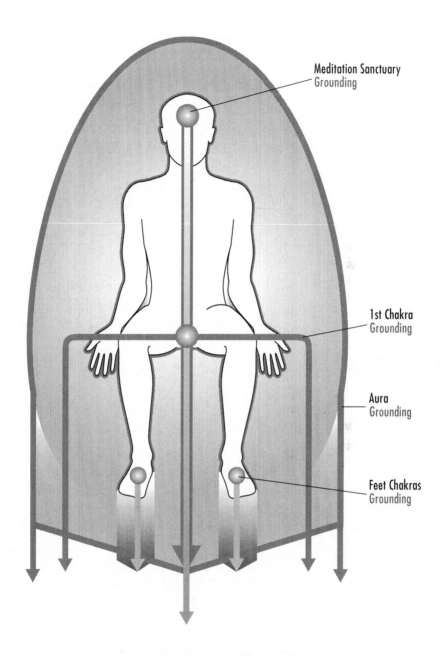

Meditation Sanctuary
Grounding

1st Chakra
Grounding

Aura
Grounding

Feet Chakras
Grounding

GROUNDING ANCHOR POINTS

difference between being ungrounded and being strongly grounded in the present. Being grounded feels good.

My observation in training sensitive people is that, once grounding is established, it brings the spirit into the body on a firm and permanent basis. When chaos strikes, you are less likely to be pushed off your center if you are grounded; you will be more able to reestablish the force field of grounding that pulls you to the earth. Being centered and grounded in your body puts you in a constant state of emotional healing and awareness. The practice of grounding gives you the option to actively alter your mood and your state of mind through affirmation and visualization. This alone is a strong prescription for health.

Here is a story from a vice president of an insurance company:

My experience shows me that it's not just active meditation that relieves stress, but also actively planting yourself in the earth. When I feel work stress or anxiety coming over me, I don't always have the luxury of taking off to meditate. However, I do have the ability to consciously ground myself. I open up my feet chakras until I feel them tingle. I let all of the stressful feelings and thoughts run through my body and out of my feet, deep into the earth. Then I work on sinking the rest of my energy through my feet and expanding it into a pyramid dug deep into the earth. At the same time, I draw up earth energy and run it through my legs and into my first chakra. I take deep breaths and focus on slowing down my body systems. With this exercise, I can become more grounded and am able to return to my work with a clearer and more objective focus.

WHAT IS GROUNDING?

Feel the aliveness in your body. That anchors you in the Now.[2]

— Eckhart Tolle

In electrical terms, grounding is a conducting connection between an electric circuit and the earth or some other conducting body. In psychological terms, grounding means to establish a feeling of self-awareness, a foundation of the consciousness of one's own self. In our energy terms, grounding means to establish an awareness of the unity of your body, mind, and spirit. How is grounding related to spirit? Our spiritual intelligence seeks a constant state of well-being, a wholeness of life. When you experience a loss of connection from the vital force of life, you are not grounded in your spiritual intelligence.

What is spiritual intelligence, and how does it relate to your intuition, wisdom, and health? Spiritual intelligence is the insight we rely upon to answers questions and solve problems. This intelligence gives meaningful direction to our lives and inspires us to transcend a methodical approach to life. We use spiritual intelligence to understand the health and healing of our body.

The practice of grounding connects you with your spiritual intelligence, which opens a cornucopia of wisdom tools for creating health and keeping you in emotional balance and harmony. To heighten this experience, visualize your spiritual intelligence as energy or light. To ground your spirit-intelligence into your body, visualize this light in the center of your head expanding straight down your body and anchoring into the earth. In this way you are affirming: "I am a spirit grounded in my body and anchored to the earth."

GROUNDING CONCEPTS

The main reason we ground a sound system is for safety. Proper grounding can prevent lethal shocks.[3]

— Trinity Sound Company

The concept of intuitive grounding involves a specific energy anatomy grounding system existing in a subtle field that connects with a person's physical anatomy. Chinese medicine provides a holistic system of health based on this principle. This energetic grounding connection allows excess or aberrant energy that enters your personal space to be released into the earth and neutralized.

The term *grounding* has different meanings in different fields. In electrical terms, a grounding circuit serves as a release valve for excess electricity. The surge protector your computer is plugged into uses such a grounding circuit; if there is a sudden burst of energy that exceeds the capacity of the computer, the surge protector directs the excess energy into the grounding circuit and down into the earth, where the energy is neutralized or grounded.

A strong grounding connection also provides a stable base from which to operate in the world. It creates a feeling of safety, centered awareness, clarity, and self-assurance. When you are grounded, your wisdom voice is clear and accessible, a natural part of your perceptional senses; your intuition walks you through the world with ease and grace.

For most people, this grounding connection is inconsistent. Some activities tend to enhance the strength of their grounding, and others tend to weaken it. What does grounding mean to you? How do you know when you are grounded? Are you grounded right now? The first step in learning to ground more consistently is to recognize the times when you are ungrounded in your life.

GROUND YOUR LIFE

Grounding your spirit, mind, and body creates a larger experience of life: more self-awareness, compassion, trust, and inner strength. All true experiences of life are an expression of health. Denial of life is a precursor to dis-ease. It is difficult to ignore life when you are a grounded person, as life roars itself present in every moment. The experience of being grounded in the present is the awareness that, no matter where you go, there you are.

When you feel disconnected from your body, mind, or spirit, what brings you back to being grounded in your intuitive intelligence? Imagine walking in a lush, green field and dropping down into the tall grass. Or imagine lying on a sunny beach and feeling the warmth of the sand. Imagine those feelings and visualize dropping all resistance from your body into the earth. Do you feel heavier, denser, and more relaxed, with an overall sensation of being pulled down to the earth? You are experiencing the pull of gravity. The constancy of nature gives us gravity as a powerful, healing force — a force that brings us back to our own center. Indeed, without gravity we would be floating off the ground!

Gravity Grounding

The mountain rests on the earth: Its position is strong only when it rises out of the earth broad and great.[4]

— The I Ching

In our quest for grounding, we have a silent, invisible, yet powerful ally: the force of gravity. We feel it all the time; it keeps our feet planted on the earth. It is a force we are often unaware of. My medical dictionary defines *gravitation* as the force of attraction by which terrestrial bodies tend to fall toward the center of the earth. In physics, gravity is the force that attracts bodies or particles of matter toward each other. Technology uses a comparable system, earthing, that relates to the live parts in electronic systems that have one or more direct connections to earth.

Simply put, we are attracted to the earth, and the earth is attracted to us. These definitions are similar to the definition of subtle energy grounding. The pull of gravity is what many people experience when they practice energy grounding.

Working with the force of gravity helps you experience and strengthen your personal grounding connection. Knowing that gravity attracts your body to the earth can support your intention to integrate energy grounding into your intuitive health practice.

At first, you may have to practice often during the day in order to experience the feeling and benefit of gravity grounding. When you have problems grounding through other means, such as visualization or intention, you may find it easier to experience a connection to the earth through gravity grounding. No matter where you are, what you are doing, or who you are with, gravity is exerting its significant force upon you.

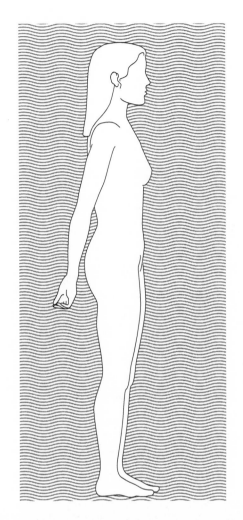

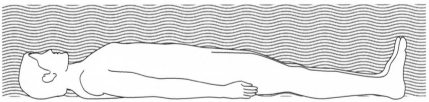

Gravity is the force that attracts terrestrial bodies to the center of the earth.
At sea level, gravity exerts 62.4 pounds of pressure per square foot.

GRAVITY GROUNDING

Your Energy Umbilical Cord

Mother is the home we come from. She is nature, soil, ocean.[5]

— Erich Fromm

The concept of Mother Earth is found in many great religions. The ancient Greeks related to the earth as a living being called Gaia. Today the idea of the earth as an organism is called the Gaia hypothesis.[6] The earth's living matter, oceans, and land surface can be described as a complex system operating as a single organism, with the capacity to sustain life; this gives the impression that the earth is a living being.[7] Ill health and dis-ease develop when something interferes with our earth grounding. This interference may be chemical, electromagnetic, spiritual, or psychological. The result is a diminished or chaotic flow of life energy through one's body, affecting one's health and well-being.

The theory of vivaxis hypothesizes that individuals establish a grounding connection to a geophysical point at birth. In other words, a person is linked with the earth via her or his own vivaxis, which is a two-way circuit. We could say that we have an invisible umbilical cord of energy attaching us to the earth via a geophysical axis of life. The grounding/vivaxis connection is a healing link for our body, which comes from and is dependent on the provisions of planet earth.[8]

Grounding healing elicits feelings of connection with life and our fellow animal kingdom. When you are grounded, you can feel and see the beauty of nature, with a sense of gratitude for being a breathing part of such a beautiful symphony.

Grounding in Daily Life

We all need to feel in balance as we go through our daily activities at home, in play, and at work. When you change activities, you will find that changing your grounding helps you maintain a healthy balance. As you move through life with your feet planted firmly on the ground, your centered attitude and emotion will affect those around you. Here is an insight on this topic from a writer who works in an advertising agency:

A breakthrough came when I started to change my grounding image fre-quently. I change it daily — sometimes even more often. Today it is a steel girder from the Golden Gate Bridge, tomorrow a chain attached to a bowl-ing ball, the next day the taproot of a tree. I now keep my balance at work by taking grounding breaks; I walk to the water cooler and back to my desk, and during those five minutes I visualize changing my grounding image. It always clears my mind so that I can focus on the task in front of me.

Grounding will also bring your highest level of integrity into your home, work, and community. When you are grounded around other people, you may find that they interact with you differently. Begin to notice how your friends, coworkers, and family respond to you when you are intentionally grounding while interacting with them.

To illustrate that point, here are two stories from corporate executives:

When I'm chairing a business meeting that seems to be going nowhere — decisions are not being made, personal verbal attacks are being made, or the talk is simply in terminal boredom mode — I reset my grounding intention to the highest level of creativity until I feel a more centered per-sonal awareness. The whole attitude of the meeting always changes to a higher productivity level.

At work, I've been using a basic grounding meditation to start all of our departmental team retreats. Starting with a meditation has become such a routine for us that everyone reminds me if I forget. We can plunge into our work, and have always had extremely focused, productive, consensual, cre-ative, and enjoyable retreats without pettiness, competitiveness, and fatigue. When it's over, everyone says they're amazed at how much we accomplished, how smoothly it flowed, and how energized they feel.

If you find yourself working with a boss or coworker who is not grounded and is creating a disharmonious workplace, your practice is to maintain your level of integrity and hold the intention that it will bring a cooperative atmosphere into your workplace. One person took that thought to work with him and came back with this report:

I went to work with the intention of not getting pushed off center by my coworkers. I knew that I had to hold onto a determined field of energy that would root me into the core of the earth. I knew I needed to do this in order to survive tension at work and not get sick. I also realized that I was getting sick because of my feelings of empathy for my coworkers' personal problems, and that attitude allowed my coworkers to ground their energy through my body. Two days of vigilant practice with my grounding technique changed my emotional attitude. I found that my grounding practice gave me more objectivity when communicating with my coworkers and more clarity about what I needed to say to them in order to get the job done. It is now normal for me to not get blown off course.

GROUNDING THROUGH VISUALIZATION, SENSATION, AND SOUND

The foolish man seeks happiness in the distance; the wise grows it under his feet.[9]

— James Oppenheim

Other tools that can help you create and maintain strong grounding connections are visualization, sensation, and sound. Together or separately, these three tools help create a stable connection with the center of the earth.

Close your eyes and imagine that you are standing inside the trunk of a giant redwood tree. You are part of the heartwood, the new wood at the center of the tree. Now visualize the trunk of that tree extending downward, deep into the center of the earth. See the roots of this great redwood encircling the earth's core, locking in and locking you in. Feel your grounding energy flowing freely down the tree's roots into the center of the earth. Feel the grounding energy of the earth flowing freely up the tree into your body. You have created a two-way grounding connection. The earth takes away energy that is out of harmony with who you are, and you receive energy from the earth that is nurturing and protective. Now add a sound by humming a pleasing tone or saying a word out loud, such as "om" or "love."

The Buddha used a combination of tools to connect with the earth for protection against the malicious forces of his adversary Mara and as a witness to his spiritual integrity. Mara attacked Buddha with frightening weapons, to which the Buddha replied in defense, "This earth is my witness." With his right hand, the Buddha touched the earth and uttered this verse:

This earth, the home of all beings,
is impartial and free of malice
toward everything which moves and does not move.
Here is the assurance that there is no deception:
take the earth as my witness.[10]

For an entire day, try to feel your grounding rather than visualizing it. Note the results; remember when it is easier and more healing for you to use the feeling of grounding as opposed to the image of grounding.

In the sections that follow, I will clarify how to recognize and use these three tools — visualization, sound, and feeling.

Grounding Energy Follows Your Visualizations

It seems that the mind has first to construct forms independently before we can find them in things.[11]

— Albert Einstein

Energy follows thought, affirmation, intention, and visualization. If you think, affirm, intend, and visualize that you are grounded, then your energy will be grounded. Visualization is an extremely powerful way to enhance your grounding.

You may already have techniques that help you feel your grounding connection with the earth, or you may be looking for new ways to experience it. Be creative; experiment with changing your grounding imagery at different times of day. Use specific visualizations that center you during exercise, public speaking, writing — whenever you want to be grounded. Here are some images to play with in your grounding meditations:

- A redwood tree

- A mountain

- A ship's anchor

- Beams of light

- An electrical cord plugged into a socket at the center of the earth

- A waterfall

- Steel beams

- A cascade of diamonds

- A pyramid, with you sitting at the top

- Niagara Falls

- Liquid terra-cotta

- A brilliant rainbow

- Two connecting magnets (you are one, the earth is the other)

You may find that certain grounding images work well for a while, and later sense that it is time to go to your grounding wardrobe and try on other images. The goal is to experience being centered and in your body all the time (or at least most of the time) so that you easily and automatically maintain the feeling and awareness of being connected to the earth. As your practice of this energy grounding progresses, you will find the process becoming easier. At first it may take repeated effort to experience being grounded. With practice, you will find that the sense of grounding comes more immediately, without effort.

Here are more images you can use to enhance your grounding connection:

- Sitting on top of a mountain

- Being within a waterfall that reaches to the center of the earth

- A ship's anchor dropping deep into the planet

- Being surrounded by a tube of golden light shining into the earth
- A whirlpool that spins in both directions, bringing your energy into the earth and the earth's energy up to you
- Lightning bolts electrically pulsing from your body into the earth
- A mud bath
- A giant drill bit
- A dragon's tail

Your imagination can supply you with limitless visualizations. Plato suggested that there was little difference between imagination and reality. He observed that anything one can reasonably imagine is eventually possible and that the plenum of imagination is the cornucopia of reality. The Sufis concluded that imagination itself is a faculty of perception; imagination leads to reality.[12] Trust your imagination as a powerful inner source.

As Einstein said, "Imagination is more important than knowledge." Unlike his contemporaries, Einstein began his experiments purely in thought, trusting his inner senses for the truths they contained. He believed "that pure thought can grasp reality, as the ancients dreamed." In his first thought experiment, he imagined the reality of light, which ultimately led him to develop his theory of relativity.[13] From pure imagination was born a revolution in science. My observation is that imagination feeds intuition, which is the language of wisdom. Wisdom is perennial, while knowledge changes. Trust your intuition and creativity to feed you new images as you need them. Practice changing your grounding visualization often.

Grounding Energy Follows Sound

Some people ground more effectively using sounds or tones. A friend and Academy alumna, Barbara Higbie is a musician and singer who does much of her energy work by using the tone of her voice or piano to set her grounding. She also senses other people's energy fields as tones, sounds, and even specific songs. Such a clairaudient person can be immediately grounded by a certain song — or instantly ungrounded by a noise or tone. Experiment with music and sound as tools to enhance your grounding. You might want to try using specific sounds, tones, or songs to assist you. If you have access to a piano or another musical instrument, try playing different notes to see which ones help you feel connected to the earth.

The association of sound with subtle energy systems is not new. In Chinese medicine, the five-element theory views the earth and the human body as linkage systems associated with musical notes.

Sound Wave Energy tapes are a uniquely designed system of sound harmonics that stimulate and balance various levels in the human energy field. One tape in the series plays a complex blend of fifty-two sonic frequencies based on the various biological elements associated with the first chakra, a major chakra associated with grounding (see the discussion of chakras in chapter 10), and its associated physiological functions. Tuning into sound frequencies allows your energy to cascade down the gravity waterfall of earth to her core.[14]

In early schools of esoteric initiation, music was used to awaken the psychic centers in specific chakras (visible to clairvoyant sight as focal points of light or glittering color). Each of these centers of force responds to a distinct musical tone, which varies with the individual. Masters of initiatory orders sang in chorus, and this volume of sound imparted its vibration to a corresponding psychic sense center, thereby accelerating its motion and heightening its powers of perception.[15]

Researchers have observed that, during mitosis, cells emit not only light but high-frequency sound. They found that it is possible to measure such ultrasonic vibrations within the body, and that often when there is light, there is also sound simultaneously. Eventually, we will be able to hear the sounds of our body by amplifying and translating them so that they become perceptible to our senses. Then we may be able to interpret those signals as one means of diagnosing illness.[16] Sound produces measurable vibratory feeling throughout the body, varying with the frequency and the amplitude of the sound used. A science called sentics is based on the ability of sound and music to induce different states of consciousness.[17]

A new kind of sound, called holophonic sound, is based on the brain's holographic way of processing sound and on the fact that human ears actually emit sound. The holophonic sound equipment's design is based on the ear-brain process, and, when wired to a computer screen, it creates a realistic, multidimensional picture using sound.[18]

"In the beginning was the word." A word is an utterance, a sonic vibrational pattern. Many hypothesize that the universe was created by sound. If that is the case, then sound is a potent force for you to use in creating a grounding connection.

Grounding Energy Follows Feeling

Meaning = Grounding + Feeling.[19]

— Steven Harnard

Another way to enhance your grounding is to *feel* that you are grounded. Become very familiar with the sensations associated with a strong grounding connection, and strive to maintain those feelings throughout the day. The "How It Feels to Be…" list in this chapter is a good starting point if you want to feel your way into a grounded connection.

Feeling is an easy way for a clairsentient person to utilize grounding somatically. You may also experiment with psychometry, using your hands to feel your connection to the earth. Sit in a chair and move your hands under your legs to gauge a subtle pressure, warmth, or tingling; this subtle energy denotes an established field of gravity grounding.

Children and Grounding

I strongly encourage parents and teachers to nurture children's innate sense of intuition. Adults often say, "Why am I learning this information about grounding now? I should have learned it in kindergarten; I wouldn't have made so many bad choices!" It is a gift to offer children a simple language for getting in touch with their feelings and to empower them with easy tools for modifying their own moods and behavior.

A mother wrote to me about an experience with her children and grounding:

> The other day while I was home, my lovely daughters got into an argument; they started to cry and get hysterical. Instead of dealing with their argument directly, I asked them to feel being grounded to the earth. They stopped crying within a couple of seconds — very unusual for my daughters, since they can be quite the drama queens. All was quiet for a little while, and then they began to argue and cry again. This time, I asked them to ground by feeling and imagining themselves being held inside Mother Earth. The argument lasted about five seconds more, then stopped for the rest of the day. Thanks for the tip!

A friend who has a child with attention deficit disorder (ADD) told me that school was not easy for her son, as he consistently had difficulty sitting down to do his homework. She found that he responded well when she helped him ground to the earth. She would stand behind him and put her hands on his shoulders, then lead him through a grounding meditation. He continued to have trouble with schoolwork, but this practice gave him the means to become independent and to feel successful no matter what his grades reflected.

An elementary school teacher told me about her experience in the classroom:

> Kids like to be grounded; it offers them a feeling of security. I've practiced grounding my students for the last twelve years. When things are chaotic or when children are having difficulty making transitions, I have them sit comfortably, close their eyes, and visualize attaching their body like an anchor into the earth. I close my eyes and guide them through a grounding meditation. It works! They get focused and ready to learn.
>
> I also have my students do some movement to get centered in their bodies. I have them stand up, and then I ask them to close their eyes while standing on one leg. It always works the same: they flail around and lose

their balance, they laugh, and then we repeat the movement on the other leg. At this point, I suggest dropping another anchor into the center of the earth. It is remarkable how controlled and balanced they are with grounding. It's short and simple, and it gets results. The noontime supervisors often remark that mine is the best class during indoor, rainy-day recesses. The truth is that a grounded group of children is best, rain or shine.

When my children were young, I would rock them to sleep while meditating. I found that if I visualized the bedroom encircled with grounded redwood trees and recalled the feeling of our favorite hiking place in Muir Woods, that would put them to sleep quickly. When I forgot to do this, they would not sleep as soundly. In fact, they would often wake up during the night.

Reflections and Journaling

This is a short integration exercise section. If you would like to assess your grounding skills, read this section now. Otherwise, you can return to it when you have time.

Reflection

Think about the items on the following lists and see if they sound familiar.

HOW IT FEELS TO BE...	
GROUNDED	**UNGROUNDED**
Peaceful	Anxious, unsure, or uneasy
Things run smoothly	Bumping into things, stubbing toes, etc.
Confident, calm, and in control	Nervous and not in control
Physically coordinated	Unable to concentrate
Mentally clear	Struggling to reach goals
Reaching goals easily	Nervous anticipation
Aware of synchronicity	Dizzy, lightheaded, spacey, overwhelmed, or confused

GROUNDED	UNGROUNDED
Feeling your energy contained in your space	In the wrong place at the wrong time
Able to move healing energy through your body	Cold feet and legs; poor circulation
Aware of yourself and your body	Lower back pain or soreness
Good inner and outer directional sense	Sciatic pains
Warm feet and legs; good circulation	Oblivious to self; without inner focus
Strong lower back	Fragmented; disassociated
Low, firm pulse in your feet and at the base of your spine	Focused exclusively on the outside world
Rooted	Everything seems difficult and effortful
Feeling in a state of gravitational flow	Easily unbalanced physically/emotionally
Deep connection to inner spirit	Low levels of joy, wisdom, or spontaneity
Sensing the nurturing energy of Mother Earth	Easily pushed out of body/head
Feeling safe being present in your body	Loss of physical/mental equilibrium
Able to handle upsets	No place for excess energy to drain out
Emotional evenness	
Enhanced self-acceptance	

Journaling

Read through the sensations in the preceding lists. Add your own entries to the lists, then count the number of items you have on your "grounded" and "ungrounded" lists. Compare the two lists.

In your journal, keep a list of personal symptoms that indicate when you are grounded and when you are not. For example, you know that you are grounded because you are calm and centered and you find it easy to default to faith rather than fear. Indications that you are ungrounded might be that you are mentally scattered and unfocused and you habitually resort to worry and fear-based thinking. Think about times in your life when you have noticed indications of being grounded. What was happening to you? What activity were you engaged in when you felt grounded? Who were you with? How about when you were ungrounded? What were you doing? Who were you with?

Using these indications, you can become more aware of your grounding. The next time you bonk your head, stub your toe, feel anxious or confused, or notice any other symptoms of being ungrounded, stop and intuit the state of your grounding. You may feel anxious and stuck in your head, with a loss of lower-body awareness. Or you may experience anxiety hunger, wherein you seek food to create a sense of weight in your body. These symptoms are reminders that you probably need to strengthen your grounding connection. Learn to notice and act on your "ungrounded" symptoms in order to integrate the benefits of grounding.

ARE YOU AWARE OF STRONG VERSUS WEAK GROUNDING?

When one tugs at a single thing in nature, he finds it attached to the rest of the world.[20]

— John Muir

More Reflections and Journaling

On the following page are lists of activities that tend to enhance or weaken grounding. Use your own intuition to assess which ones apply to you. As you become more aware of your grounding, some of the activities that tend to unground you will no longer do so.

Reflection

Look at the following lists of activities and reflect on their implications in your life.

ACTIVITIES AND THINGS THAT...	
ENHANCE GROUNDING	**WEAKEN GROUNDING**
Physical activities: walking, running, biking, etc.	Sedentary activities
Being in nature; being around animals	Watching television, especially news reports
Massage; bodywork	Being indoors for extended periods
Being around grounded people	Driving in heavy traffic
Being with people who respect you	Stress or pain
A nutritious diet	Being around ungrounded, unstable people
A fulfilling career	Being with people who control you
Artistic expression	A nutritionally deficient diet; alcohol; sugar
Grounding meditation	Working at a job you dislike
Pressing your feet into the earth	Boredom
Opening your foot chakras	Ungrounding meditation
Humor and joy	Mean-spirited remarks; cowardice; anger
	Lack of sleep

Journaling

Think about the activities and things in the preceding lists. Add to these lists from your experience, then count the number of items on your "enhance grounding" and "weaken grounding" lists. Compare the two lists.

How do the "enhance" and "weaken" lists compare to your experience of your grounding? Are there activities on one list that you would switch to the other? What activities can you add to the lists? Who tends to uproot your grounding connection? And who allows you to remain grounded? Take a moment to think about these things and write about them in your journal. Keep this list in a place where you will look at it daily. This will help you become more aware of your grounding and the situations that affect it.

I hope that this chapter on grounding has given you at least one piece of healthy-living information to think about and healing prescriptions that you can immediately use to bring more balance and energy into your life. Do not limit yourself in your grounding practice. You may discover other tools that work for you!

Go to the next chapter, "The Grounding Meditation Practice," when you feel ready to apply the grounding thoughts from this chapter to meditations, affirmations, and tips on how to live every day with a greater connection to the earth.

Chapter 5

THE GROUNDING MEDITATION PRACTICE

The regular practice of meditation is the single most powerful means of increasing intuition.

— Frances Vaughan

*N*ow is the time to put into practice the core intuitive health tool of grounding. This is an integral item in your Intuition Medicine toolbox and the foundation upon which you will build all the other intuitive skills that follow in this book. I would suggest that you read through this chapter completely before you begin the practices described in it.

This chapter has six separate sections, covering the contemplative, observational, daily-living, experimental, affirmation-setting, and introspective practices of grounding. You may find that you prefer one of these modes of practice — the affirmations, for example — or maybe a combination will appeal to you, such as contemplative meditations and journal writing. Experiment with what works for you at this stage in your development; you will probably try all six grounding modes eventually, and naturally integrate what feels right to you as a personal practice. As you take the time to develop and become fluent in the language of intuition, you are reclaiming a vital human sense.

Contemplative Meditations

The focus of these grounding meditations is to give you a simple and powerful tool that centers you in your body and connects your body with the earth. Grounding meditation is an inherent part of the healthy, living practice of Intuition Medicine, but it may take repetition to fully integrate constant grounding as a contemplative and eventually as a practical skill.

The grounding meditations are long, so I suggest that you read one and then close your eyes and let your intuition guide you to follow whatever piece of the meditation you recall best for short, five- to fifteen-minute meditations. Which piece you concentrate on may change each time you do this, or it may stay as a constant contemplative focus of your meditation practice. You may choose to do these meditations one after the other, or you can do each alone. After doing a meditation, you may want to take time to reflect on your experiences, or you might want to read the post-meditation questions and write notes on your personal reflections in your journal. Do what works for you; there is no one right way to do the meditation practice.

I offer you two contemplative grounding meditations. The first is a prone gravity-grounding meditation to use for body relaxation and stress release. The lower Gravity Grounding illustration on page 46 shows a figure in the prone position for the sake of this meditation, however, you may and should also practice gravity grounding while you stand, walk, and run and in other positions. The second can be done in a seated position and focuses on developing connections between your body and spirit — your emotional and spiritual intelligences.

Prone Gravity-Grounding Meditation

- Find a comfortable place to lie down. Close your eyes and begin to breathe slowly, inhaling through your nose and exhaling through your mouth. Breathe with the intention of slowing down and relaxing. Focus on listening to the sound of your breath. Do this for about a minute. Then let your breathing return to its natural rhythm.

- Come into communication with yourself by bringing your attention into your head and resting your attention at the area of your hypothalamus gland, which is located in the center of your head. We will call this place your meditation sanctuary — your sacred, quiet space of self-reflection and the intuitive spot for sensing your inner voice of wisdom. (See the Meditation Sanctuary illustration on page 75.) Greet yourself and hear, sense, and feel the presence of your inner voice. I suggest that you actually say hello to yourself mentally to establish a ritual for coming into sacred space.

- Within your meditation sanctuary, evoke a feeling of being surrounded by nature. Draw upon a favorite place at the beach, in the woods, on top of a mountain, or near a river. Recall a place you know in nature that stimulates a familiar sensation of peace and tranquility. Be in the center of the memory of that serene experience, and affirm the presence of that sacred outer place as your inner meditation sanctuary. Be there. Be in a no-think place. Hold that feeling and energy for a quiet minute.

- Focus on the feeling that your nature-memory stimulates — a whole-body sensation of peace and tranquility. Feel the elemental force of the earth; sense the force of gravity, the energy that attracts bodies toward the center of the earth. Notice how your body feels. Feel the force of gravity sinking you down into Mother Earth. Sense the pressure that gravity applies to your whole body. Affirm that you are relaxing your body, letting go of any resistance, and dropping into the force field of gravity. Take a deep breath and relax. Hold that feeling of gravity grounding for a moment.

- Beginning at your head, move through each body part and sense any energy blocks, tension, or stress. When you locate a disharmonious energy, focus on that area and visualize the force of gravity pulling the disharmonious energy out of your body and down into the earth.

- Scan your head, eyes, ears, nose, mouth, and chin. Sense any points of stress or tension. See the areas of light or dark energy. Locate any pain or inner noise. Put your attention on each area of discomfort and feel the force of gravity moving the energy block or pain down and out of your body and sinking it into the earth.

- Now focus on your neck, shoulders, arms, and hands. Sense any areas of tension, stress, pain, or blocked energy patterns. Feel the force of gravity directing any discomfort out of your neck, shoulders, arms, and hands and dropping it straight down into the earth. Take a deep breath and relax these areas of your body. Notice any sensations of temperature change, tingling, or muscle relaxation.

- Next, focus on your back, from your neck down to your buttocks. Feel any aches, pain, or tense muscles; perceive any areas of blocked energy. Begin to slowly and gently visualize gravity dissolving and releasing the uncomfortable feelings and washing them down into the earth. Let go of the energy. Breathe into this area of your body, relax, and sense your whole body being pulled down into the earth.

- Now pay attention to your upper torso: your chest and solar plexus. Feel any tense muscles and pained areas. Sense areas of dark or congested energy. Begin to direct the force of gravity through these areas and release any unpleasant feelings down into the earth.

- Now focus on your pelvis, back and front. Scan this area by feel, using your inner vision and knowing perception. Feel the force of gravity cleansing out any blocked energy and flushing it down into the earth.

- Focus on your legs: thighs, knees, calves, feet, and toes. Notice tension, pain, and energy blocks. Drop any discomfort from your legs and release it down into the earth.

- Trust your intuition and know the areas in your body that are calling for a cleansing release. Focus on each area and flush the discordant energy down and out of your body into the ground. Spend a couple of minutes scanning for any out-of-balance energy in your body and grounding it off.

- Bring your attention into your meditation sanctuary and greet yourself. Sense the force of gravity moving through your meditation sanctuary with the intention of clearing out all energy that takes you out of communication with yourself.

- Be present now in that inner, quiet, still place. Hold that feeling for a moment.

- From that point of perception, sense your whole body, from the top of your head to your toes. Feel the force of gravity pulling your entire body down into the force field of the earth. Drop your energy low to the ground and feel your entire body holding that grounding connection to Mother Earth. Hold that meditation feeling for one minute.

Seated Grounding Meditation

- Sit in a comfortable chair with your feet flat on the ground, your back straight, and your arms and hands in a resting position.

- Come into communication with yourself by centering your attention in your meditation sanctuary. Breathe slowly and gently. Make this focus the most important thing you are doing now. Breathe out any distracting thoughts or sounds and gently bring your attention back to your breathing. Focus on your breathing for one minute.

- With your attention in your meditation sanctuary, visualize the energy of your spirit as a color, symbol, or knowing; experience the energy of yourself as spirit. Visualize a current of your spiritual energy moving from the center of your meditation sanctuary and running vertically through your body down to the center of the earth. Visualize anchoring your spirit through your body into Mother Earth. See and feel your spirit coming more fully into your body. (See the Grounding Anchor Points illustration on page 41.)

- Greet your body, drop your emotional energy low to the ground, and feel the slow, dense resonance of the force field of the earth. Sense the pulse of the planet — the heartbeat of Mother Earth. This rhythmic pulsation is the earth's electromagnetic force field, which continuously bathes our bodies with a natural healing current.

- Put your attention on your first chakra, which is located at the base of your spine. Call forth an image that represents your emotional grounding. Trust the first insight you receive. Visualize that emotional grounding symbol connecting organically from the base of your spine and dropping an anchor down to the center of the earth. Create an inner-earth connector for this symbol to hook into. Feel the pull of gravity on your whole body. Visualize this emotional grounding expanding as wide as your body and pulling your whole body down into the core of the earth. Hold that feeling for a moment.

- Bring your attention down to your feet chakras, located at the bottom of your feet. Visualize them opening up like a flower. Feel the pulse of the earth in your feet. Visualize planting your feet into the earth. Practice keeping your feet chakras open all the time to enhance your connection to the earth so that you may walk through the world with ease and grace.

- Refocus your attention in your meditation sanctuary and take a deep inhale-and-exhale breath. Focus on your whole body. Sense and see any areas where blocked energy is located. Scan for unhealthy energy areas: frozen or congested light, dark or murky colors, or any symbol or presence that you feel is not in harmony with your well-being.

- Visualize the force of gravity pulling on each negatively charged area, magnetically drawing all unhealthy energy away from that location, and running that energy down to the core of the earth.

Visualize a release valve or tube that allows the energy a free-fall space to run down. Practice releasing the negative energy and letting it go.

- Come into communication with yourself by greeting yourself with your inner voice. From the center of your meditation sanctuary, reaffirm your grounding connection to the earth. See and feel your spiritual energy from the center of your sanctuary, and visualize a current of yourself as spirit running through your body and connecting into the center of the earth.

- Drop your emotional energy low to the ground again. Put your attention on your first chakra, visualize your emotional grounding symbol, and see that symbol expanding as wide as your body as you visualize it moving down to the core of the earth. This grounds your emotional body.

- Be in the center of your meditation sanctuary. Hold this grounding meditation for one minute.

Observational Practice: Journaling

You will get the most from this introspective practice section if you write all the questions and your responses to them in a journal. Answering the questions immediately after completing a contemplative meditation is the best way to integrate the experience.

Before writing in your journal, take a moment to reflect on some general questions: How does it feel to be grounded? This may be a different sensation than you are used to. Do you like it? Is it comfortable? It may actually take some time to get used to the feelings of being grounded, but once you are accustomed to it, you will wonder how you ever functioned without grounding.

Post-Meditation Questions

Now take a few moments to consider the following questions:

1. Were you able to sense your grounding connection?

2. Describe the feelings that accompanied your experience.

3. When have you felt this way before? What activities or events have triggered a grounded feeling within you?

4. Quickly scan the list of grounding visualizations found on page 51 in chapter 4 and, using your intuition, get a sense of which of those images will help you to maintain a strong grounding connection. What other visualizations can you add to the list?

5. From your own experience can you add other situations or activities to the list of grounding and ungrounding events you began in chapter 4?

6. Can you add other symptoms and sensations of grounding to your list? (See "'When to Dial Down' or 'Open Up' Your Chakras" in appendix 2.)

Daily-Living Tips

- During the day, pause often to notice the state of your grounding.

- As needed, utilize gravity, visualizations, knowing, or other tools to strengthen your grounding.

- Become aware of activities, locations, and people that tend to unground you.

- Become aware of activities, locations, and people that enhance your grounding.

Experiments: Try This!

- You can experience the power of gravity grounding in the bathtub. Next time you take a bath, do not get out of the tub when you pull the plug. Instead, lie there as the water drains out. You will be treated to a very tactile sense of gravity's power. Human bodies are naturally buoyant, so water reduces the effect gravity has on us. If you have been soaking in water for at least twenty minutes, you will have a sense of being glued to the bottom of the tub when the water is gone. Enjoy! That is the feeling of gravity grounding — and that is the feeling you can create in your energy system all the time.

- When you wake up in the morning and step out of bed, focus on your breathing. Pay attention to feeling gravity grounding descending to your legs and feet until they start to tingle and warm up. Next, jump into a hot shower and stand there with your eyes closed, feeling the water running from the top of your head down to your toes. Use this morning meditation ritual to remind your body to connect to the earth. During the day, if you feel that your emotional grounding is weak, take a long drink of cool water and remind your body to feel that water grounding you into the earth.

Affirmations: Repeat Often

- I know my spirit.

- I respect my body.

- I bring my body and spirit together often in loving friendship.

- I walk with my feet on the ground.

- I trust my insights and sensitivities.

- I know myself.

- I practice the art of spiritual integrity.

- I am guided by my intuitive intelligence.

- I listen to my inner wisdom voice.

- I walk through the world with ease and grace.

Trust

Congratulations on taking a giant step forward through grounding on your intuitive-wisdom, spiritual-intelligence journey. Your ability to walk through this world in a grounded, centered manner will assist you in accessing the wisdom of your intuitive intelligence.

As you learn to trust your intuition just as you trust your sight, smell, taste, touch, and hearing, you will begin to recognize the abundance of information it offers. With focus and practice, your intuition will become the most utilized of your six senses.

Chapter 6

MEDITATION SANCTUARY:
MEDITATION IS A LOCATION

The idea of a sacred place where walls and laws of the temporal world may dissolve to reveal a wonder is as old as the human race.

— Joseph Campbell

*T*rue meditation occurs in the Now, and the core of most meditation practices lies in making ourselves present in the moment. Meditation can be defined as healing through inner sources. By contrast, medication involves healing through external sources. But how do you locate "Now"? When do you know that you are in that place of presence? In this chapter, I introduce you to a location that I call the meditation sanctuary. This is an inner place you may go during meditation and also a place you can choose to live in full-time. This new place of living gives you a mystic's perspective on life. It provides a quiet inner sanctum and a constant state of inner peace. The meditation sanctuary is the human harbor where your spirit grounds within your body to experience present time. In the book *The Power of Now*, Eckhart Tolle says, "You cannot be in your body without being intensely in the present moment."[1] Tolle describes the Now as the main portal through which one is intensely aware of the present moment. To find that location, one must cease constant mental activity. Tolle describes meditation as a simple way to stop mental commentary so that one may enter the portal of the present moment. In my experience, grounding in one's body is a prerequisite to experiencing the Now state of meditation.

THE NOW

For us convinced physicists the distinction between past, present, and future is an illusion, though a persistent one.[2]

— Albert Einstein

It might seem odd to talk about an intangible concept like Now as an actual place. Many who meditate experience the Now as a "moving present."[3] In fact, there is no equation that can prove the existence of a present moment. Science lacks many equations and measurement instruments for nonphysical phenomena that intelligent people experience as life-transforming. Recently, astrophysicists have discovered that what appears to be empty space in the sky is a tangible, measurable occurrence in our universe. When you look into the night sky, you see the lights of the stars scattered amidst what your mind tells you is dark nothingness. But this "nothing," called dark matter, is now known to be filled with something.[4] Newly engineered instruments are finding this dark matter to be measurable and present in empty space, calling it a "Universal Web."[5] As well as transforming our understanding of time and space, these instruments may also be able to measure the subtle human energy field.

THE PLACE OF NOW

Time is pliable and subjective.[6]

— Itzhak Bentov

Your pathway to the Now is a practice of meditation. In meditation, you can verify the existence of the Now with your intuitive, sensitive body.

Within your head, you can also locate the "power of Now" in the area of your hypothalamus gland. Neurochemist Candace Pert, PhD, has researched and tested this temporal portal and found it to be an organ of intuition.7 For many years, I theorized, based both on direct experience and years of clinical observation, that the hypothalamus is the "motherboard" of intuition in the body.

It is also noteworthy that the hypothalamus relates to emotional addiction, and addictive emotions remove a person from the spiritual realm and the Now. The movie *What the Bleep Do We Know?!* offers an explanation of the tendency to cling to unhealthy mental attitudes. For example, in the mental attitude of a "victim personality," the hypothalamus produces "victim" amino acids that flood the body, carrying bundles of past victim-story emotions. If a person stops thinking and feeling habitual victim-oriented thoughts, the hypothalamus stops putting out these amino acids and the person goes into withdrawal. This is why it can be so difficult to let go of painful memories; it takes a lot of work!

If you have trouble releasing victimhood or painful memories, there is hope. During your meditation sanctuary practice, you can flood your body with healthy emotions by repeating positive affirmations. In time, this will hardwire a healthier emotional reality into your body. This is a powerful practice for creating a body of health.

The hypothalamus is more than just a delivery system for emotions; we have inner and outer sight because of it. When light enters the eye, it travels to the vision centers of the brain and to the hypothalamus, which controls almost all the functions of the pituitary, which in turn affects all the endocrine glands. This means that the hypothalamus is a major collecting and controlling station for information from the external and internal environment.8

The hypothalamus consists of concentrated bundles of neuronal fibers within a vacuum. These neurons act as transducers — devices that are actuated by power from one system and supply power, usually in another form, to a second system — that use quantum electromagnetic effects depending on the polarizing ability of the vacuum. The vacuum itself becomes a transducer into physical state-energies for consciousness-energy in nonphysical states. The vacuum is the physically effective yet nonphysical transition state that leads to and from the domains of consciousness. This implies that the hypothalamus is a bioenergetic mechanism for dissolving time-concepts in order to explore timeless metadimensions.[9]

Energy healer Barbara Brennan, author of *Hands of Light*, teaches a "high sense perception" program that includes visualizing a meditation spot that she describes as a beautiful point of light in the center of the head that grows into a brilliant ball of light.[10] She clairvoyantly sees this light as being located in the root area of the crown and third-eye chakras, where the pituitary and pineal glands are located (see the Meditation Sanctuary illustration on page 75 and the Endocrine System and Chakra Correspondences illustration on page 146). This corresponds to my theory that intuitive perception is located in the hypothalamus area. As my realtor friends say, "Location is everything." And, indeed, in order to develop your intuition pragmatically and contemplatively, you must bring your awareness into your meditation sanctuary, that private, sacred space within yourself that is an entryway to the experience of the Now.

"NO TIME" AND THE NOW

The body is always in time; the spirit is always in timelessness.[11]

— Aldous Huxley

The possible nonexistence of time has been discussed by many people, from Einstein all the way up to contemporary quantum theorists. Numerous books have been devoted to the idea that linear time does not exist. One theory argues that instants of time are distinct entities that should not be thought of as joined in a linear sequence: this is a scientific definition of the intuitive theory of time as a nonlocal, present-now experience that I am presenting.[12] This concept, that the reality of the universe is made up of instants of time, textures a richly structured world made of Nows.[13] Meditation provides us with a portal to that deeper reality, creating a sense that time is entangled within timelessness. Our access to the past is only through memories and records, which are in fact present-time phenomena.[14] Our perception of history, time, and space is relative to the

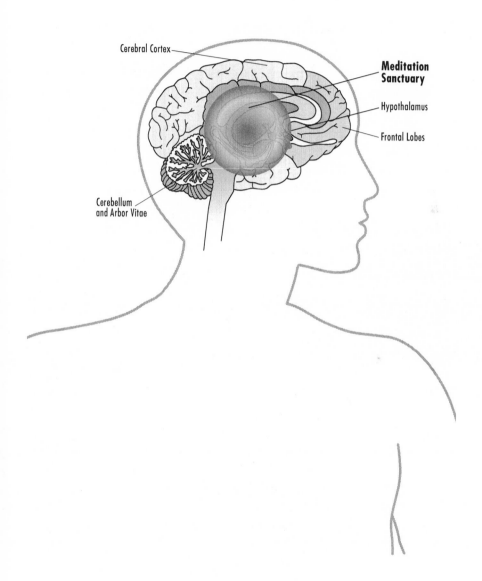

Cerebral Cortex

Meditation Sanctuary

Hypothalamus

Frontal Lobes

Cerebellum and Arbor Vitae

MEDITATION SANCTUARY

experience of the Now. As Einstein's theory of relativity posits, everything is happening now. With present-time meditation practice, your perception of time changes. A second-year Intuition Medicine practitioner shared his experience of the benefits of the practice:

> *When I am in my meditation sanctuary, I notice that my jaw and brow relax, my shoulder tension unknots, and my focus is more present on what I am doing. My mind slows down, and quietness descends through my entire body. I am able to connect with my spirit. I no longer dwell on past scenarios or fear the future. The quality of time changes; there's a clarity and stillness to what I am experiencing. I feel responsive to the world without worry, fear, fretting, or anxiety. I feel right in the moment.*

In an altered state of consciousness, such as meditation, our perception of time changes; so-called subjective time becomes longer and reaches infinity as consciousness expands.[15] Buddhist philosophy identifies three types of time: "profane time" (in which there is no awareness of an active spiritual ingredient), "grand time" (in which time is shaped by cycles, patterns, and myths), and "no time" (an experience beyond time). "Timelessness" is the Western term closest to "no time." You have probably experienced timelessness in ordinary moments, such as when gardening, working creatively, listening to music, playing sports, or walking in nature. People usually experience this as a feeling of serenity, deep silence, and everything fading away and a sense of eternity. These experiences of timelessness, of the Now, are inside you.[16]

BE HERE NOW

I'm late, I'm late for a very important date. No time to say hello, goodbye. I'm late, I'm late, I'm late.[17]

— Lewis Carroll

What would you do if you had more time? Where would you travel if you could move into the past and future? On January 27, 1995, American and British scientists conducting investigations in Antarctica noticed a spinning gray fog in the sky over the South Pole. They initially believed that it was an ordinary storm, but it didn't change form or move directionally. The researchers launched a weather balloon into the fog to register its wind speed, temperature, and moisture. But the weather balloon soared upward and immediately disappeared. The researchers manually retrieved the weather balloon and checked its instruments. They were extremely surprised to see that a chronometer in the weather balloon displayed the date of January 27, 1965 — the same day, but thirty years earlier. After verifying that the instrumentation was in good working order, they repeated the experiment several times; each time, the chronometer displayed the same time in the past. They called this phenomenon "the time gate."[18]

Einstein's theory of a space-time continuum states that the apparent linearity of events depends on the observer. Our past lives may be happening right now in a different space-time continuum. Many of us have experienced past lives and feel their effects as if they were a short time ago. But rarely do we speak of how our future lives are affecting the life we are experiencing right now.

Time is a form of energy that accomplishes things or allows phenomena to occur. As time develops into physical reality, it injects the world with new properties of creation. Time is enigmatic; it appears immediately everywhere. The altered properties of a certain second of time appear instantaneously everywhere at once, just as time is everywhere. Time has "density" properties that have been studied in an astrophysical laboratory using gyroscopes, asymmetrical pendulums, and torsion balance instruments. The results showed that time is thinner near the sender of an action and denser near the receiver. This demonstrates a decrease in time-density near the cause and an increase of time-density near the effect.[19]

As we live our lives in the Now, it is possible that we are rewriting our personal histories, both present and future.[20] Psychological experiments are exploring the possibility that the mind is in contact with its own future state or, alternately, that it is slightly "spread out" in time.[21]

BACK TO THE FUTURE

Do not dwell in the past, do not dream of the future; concentrate the mind on the present moment.[22]

— Buddha

Evidence suggests that we can get specific, meaningful information from anywhere or "anywhen." The future may not be the only thing that can be formed and reshaped by human thought. A theory proposed by Princeton University aerospace engineer Robert Jahn suggests that, just as a photon is both a particle and a wave, perhaps consciousness also has complementary states. In ordinary states, the mind is more particlelike and is firmly localized in space and time. This perception is supported by the ordinary subjective experience of being an isolated, independent creature. But in unusual, nonordinary states of awareness, our minds may be more wavelike and no longer localized in space or time. This observation is supported by subjective experiences of timelessness, mystical unity, and intuition.

According to Einstein's theory of space-time and other recent time theories, the universe is fundamentally interconnected because we are all constructed of the same "stuff." This may be why, in meditation, we are able to directly experience the past, present, and future as the Now.[23]

Parapsychology researchers Marilyn Schlitz and Helmut Schmidt conducted laboratory experiments on psychokinesis (mental interaction with animate or inanimate matter), which proved their hypothesis — "Mental thought can affect inanimate objects." However, to their surprise, the experiment also demonstrated that the mind can reach back through time and affect the past. In this study, cassette recordings of one hundred random tones, some pleasing and some just bursts of noise, no two tapes alike, were mailed to test subjects. The subjects were told to listen to the tapes and attempt to psychokinetically increase the duration of the pleasing sounds and decrease the duration of the noise. After the subjects completed the task, Schlitz and Schmidt compared copies of each of the original recording tapes, which had not left the laboratory, with the copies that were returned from the test subjects in order to investigate the before-and-after effects. They discovered that the subjects were successful in altering the tapes that they had listened to. When they checked the original, control laboratory tapes for comparative analysis, they discovered that the control tapes now also contained longer stretches of pleasing sounds than of noise, making them similar to the test subjects' altered tapes. In other words, it appeared that the subjects had psychokinetically reached back through time and affected the randomized process through which their cassettes had been made. This experiment was not hypothesizing that the present could affect the past, so the results were truly unexpected and surprising.[24]

Schlitz and Schmidt also discovered that subjects who were regular meditators exerted a greater effect on the tape recordings than nonmeditators did, suggesting that contact with the unconscious is a key to accessing reality-structuring. If the past is not frozen, time is an illusion, and reality is a mental creation, then the possibilities of human potential expand to infinity.

YOU PERCEIVE YOUR OWN REALITY

Unfortunately, no one can be told what the Matrix is. You have to see it for yourself. This is your last chance. After this, there is no turning back. You take the blue pill, the story ends. You wake up in your bed and believe whatever you want to believe. You take the red pill, you stay in Wonderland, and I show you how deep the rabbit hole goes. Remember, all I'm offering is the truth. Nothing more.[25]

— Morpheus to Neo in *The Matrix,* by Andy and Larry Wachowski

Psychology, psychiatry, and hard science are combined in the work of aerospace engineer Robert Jahn and psychologist Brenda Dunne in their Princeton Engineering Anomalies Research (PEAR) laboratory. Their research is validating what mystics have always known: The world is not static, and the forces of human perception influence reality as much as geophysical and cosmological forces do. Twenty years of highly credible results in the PEAR laboratory have shown that perception has a measurable influence on matter and reality.[26] So, it is clearly beneficial that you understand how to use your perceptual ability to create a positive, healthful, joy-filled life.

Entanglement — the defining trait of quantum theory, which Einstein dubbed "spooky action at a distance" — has opened up a new realm of reality through demonstrations in laboratory experiments that two microscopic particles can instantaneously affect each other at a distance. Physicists now believe that this entanglement exists everywhere, all the time, and that it also affects the wider macroscopic world we live in. Researchers are calling this phenomenon "quantum weirdness" and "spooky interaction," and theorize that it enables us to retain control in our everyday world at a physical level. More "quantum magic" theory suggests that particles can also be entangled across time; some experiments show that the future can influence the past, challenging our previous understanding of cause and effect. This instantaneous causality puts time on equal footing with space in quantum theory. In other words, time — like space — is a measurable equation in our universe.[27] One way of understanding this is to imagine the universe as one piece of fabric woven together by entangled strings of time and space. In this model, when you pull one of the strings, there is a simultaneous effect through the entire warp of the string that changes the form of the entire fabric, no matter where the original string that was pulled is located.

What does this mean in the mystical realm? It corroborates the sayings that "energy follows your thoughts" and "you create your reality." Entanglement theory gives intellectual substance to the concepts of perception, visualization, and intention.

Perception is a creative force, empowered through visualization, knowing, and intention. Visualization is a way to use imagination to gain intuitive insight, with imagery serving as the language of intuition.[28] Knowing provides the insight to see through the filtering screen of thoughts, images, and feelings to the formless context of knowledge.[29] Intention is a deliberate decision to create. It is premeditated; it is planned. Intention is not a fleeting thought. It is not a wish, hope, or worry. It is a decision, made with purpose, to produce something. It is a force unto itself.[30] When your awareness is focused in the hypothalamus, you are operating from a place of fluidity, effectiveness, and calm assurance. You are truly smarter because you generate a state of mind in which your intellectual analysis of a situation is combined with acute sensory perception and creative intuition.[31]

THE HEALTH PRACTICE OF MEDITATION

The secret of health for both mind and body is not to mourn for the past, not to worry about the future, or not to anticipate troubles, but to live in the present moment wisely and earnestly.[32]

— Buddha

The alchemy of spirit is in a state of rapid expansion. Through eons of development, we have evolved human bodies that now include the subtle system of energy anatomy. Human evolution is characterized and limited by the penetration of spirit into dense body matter. Spirituality is defined as the feelings, thoughts, experiences, and behaviors that arise from a search for that which is generally considered sacred or holy. Spirituality is usually, though not universally, considered to involve a sense of connection with an absolute, immanent, or transcendent spiritual force, however named, as well as the conviction that meaning, value, direction, and purpose are valid aspects of the universe. Consciousness is the capacity to react to, attend to, and be aware of self and other. Consciousness subsumes all categories of experience, including perception, cognition, intuition, instinct, will, and emotion, at all levels.[33] The more spirit that is present in body matter, the higher is the consciousness of the entity. The entity applies that consciousness, through its focused intentionality, in the various acts of daily life.[34] Through the practice of intentional meditation, transformational changes occur in both the body and spirit.

Meditation practice alters your vision, both physically and spiritually. Ocular vision requires more than a functioning physical organ (the eyes). Without an inner light, we are blind. As Arthur Zajonc says, "The light of the mind must flow into and marry with the light of nature to bring forth a world"[35] — a world that becomes our reality. So it is with all of our five physical senses. Whatever our current reality is, and whatever meaning we attribute to it, it can be altered by changing the focus of our attention and intention, thereby changing our life. Meditation practice in the Now moves us to encompass expanded vistas of reality.[36]

During meditation practice, many people begin to experience light within their meditation sanctuary. This seems to be the seed kernel that brings light to and develops the energy body into a more advanced organ, which begins to perceive and thus interact with reality beyond the physical world. With practice, sensitivity to the intuitive world develops. As Barbara Brennan says about the effect of meditation practice, "We are each living transformation systems. We are truly spiritualizing matter."[37]

Intuitive perception has heightened in relationship to the morphological changes in our human systems. Those of us who are attuned to spiritual alchemy find in the evolving nature of spirit within matter an invitation to communicate to a larger audience about the mystical nature of human beings — aspects of ourselves that have mostly been shared in secret societies and codified in symbols. It is time for initiation into the birthright of the language of intuition. Meditation practice is the initiation ritual. Spiritual wisdom is found in the quiet, still Now of meditation.

ARE YOU IN THE PRESENT?

Let us not look back in anger or forward in fear, but around in awareness.[38]

— Black Elk

Healthy emotions are located in the present; even reflections on the past or future are possible to hold as present thoughts. You can quickly self-diagnose in the present, as you are able to immediately sense the first signs of dis-ease and choose to make a healing change. Repressed anger is an emotion that pollutes health and is easy enough to change into cleansing anger, expressed with right thought and an objective perspective. Anger can be transformed by communicating your feelings while holding your perception in present time. The following story illustrates this concept; it is an account by a meditation practitioner who became physically sick while going through divorce proceedings:

I practice being present in my life — for good reasons. I am able to express so much more of who I am, as I am not scared of other people's reactions anymore. I am not only able to stay present when somebody feels anger, but I am also able — for the first time in my life — to feel my own anger and express it authentically. I have gotten to know myself much better in terms of my needs and wants, and I am able to truly listen to and take care of my body. When I listen to my intuition and follow through with the directions from my inner voice, I can heal my hurt feelings faster and I know how to take care of my physical disease. My experience of being in the world is safer and healthier now that I am truly here, feeling the present.

The present moment is a place of power, life, and depth. It is a rich space/time filled with a cornucopia of human health. It is the doorway to other realms, other foci of consciousness — the gateway to intuition.

PRACTICE STAYING IN THE NOW

Synchronicity: A coincidence in time. A simultaneous matching of inner unconscious or conscious thoughts with synchronized timing and manifestation in the outer world.[39]

— Carl Jung

Your choices in life are endless when you live in the present. The ability to influence all aspects of your life comes from within. You might find that paying attention to your immediate process — really being present with yourself — is at first a challenge and an emotional stretch. Present-time perception is a practice of being neutral and objective with yourself and others. When you act with focused objectivity and do not take things personally, the action and outcome produce less angst, worry, and regret, and situations work out for the greater good. Being in the moment enhances your personal relationships, as you can be more objective and present with a person, with less concern for the outcome. You can clearly choose to walk away from situations that do not serve you and others, and tolerance and forgiveness will come more easily. A spirit grounded and present in a body is the most powerful engine for healing and change.

A thirty-year-old woman who is a legal assistant wrote this reflection about being in the present:

Living in present time has helped me find peace with an old friend. Before I began meditating regularly, we couldn't have a conversation without me trotting out past hurts, and that caused huge amounts of pain. I was always feeding the fire that made me miserable. I was starting to think that nothing would take away my hurt and anger at him. But then I began my meditation sanctuary practice. I'm sure he thinks it's a miracle that I've stopped torturing him with stories of everything he ever did that I felt badly about. I now see him in the present, rather than as who he was in the past. It's a challenge to be present all the time, but I can see that it is a happier, more productive place to be.

MEDITATION SANCTUARY PERCEPTION ENHANCES SIGHT AND THOUGHT

Every time you don't follow your inner guidance, you feel a loss of energy, a loss of power, a sense of spiritual deadness.[40]

— Shakti Gawain

During your daily activities, you will know that you are in your meditation sanctuary when your peripheral ocular vision quietly widens; you may have increased depth perception even in darkness. In decision-making and daily tasks, you will rely less on frontal-brain thinking; rationality and analysis will cease to be the dominant inner voice.

When you meditate with your eyes closed, you will experience an inner sense of 360-degree perception. Your quieter intuitive inner voice will gain credence. Your spiritual life will become part of your pragmatic affairs, woven through the fabric of your day. Although our minds acquire information in an inherently subjective fashion, Western culture teaches us to conceptualize and express our experience and activity primarily via precise "this, not that" objective discriminations, largely neglecting the intangible subjective dimensions that can blur those distinctions.[41] Socrates called the inner voice the daimon (Divine); William James used the term noetic (direct knowing); and Plato described the soul's remembrance of truth as anamnesis.[42]

The practice of transpersonal psychology values spiritual insights as healing therapy. This approach presents a much-needed perspective on trusting insight and inner knowing and limits the role of analytical processing in therapy. It can take the analytical mind years or lifetimes to accomplish what can be accomplished in a few seconds by a person who listens to the inner voice and perceives information via the meditation sanctuary.

Here is a relevant comment from an attorney who has been practicing Intuition Medicine for three years:

One of the biggest hurdles I face in doing energy work and self-healing is my tendency to rely on "rational," logical thought. I certainly can't blame this tendency on my legal education or my being a practicing attorney. It is a spot from which I have primarily operated since childhood. I spent years in traditional therapy attempting to solve my problems through rational thinking, in the process twisting myself into intellectual pretzels in an effort to heal past traumas. It is interesting to note that figuring out personal puzzles in traditional talk therapy, while intellectually appealing, was not healing per se. At best, rational thought was a helpful companion. At its worst, the analytical mind was a roadblock to healing. I find now that my inner intelligence — intuition — feeds me with soul-filled information that I can move into energy, which in turn has a potent healing effect on my body. It also takes the emotional charge out of my trauma-filled memories.

PRACTICAL MEDITATION IN DAILY LIFE

Time is a form of energy! It is to time's properties that we should look in order to find the source that maintains the phenomenon of life in the world.[43]

— Nikolai Kozyrez

Your meditation practice sets the warp through which your spiritual life can be woven during your day. When you meditate regularly, you get what you need when you need it; life comes in unexpected forms and is exactly what you need at any given moment. In life, unexpected things happen. Shifts occur that you cannot always prepare for. When time is still and you are present with the experience of the moment, you are imperturbable, unflappable, and hyperconnected to your knowingness and authenticity. The decisions you make will flow easily and effortlessly. You will speak the truth from the center of the Now with an authentic voice. The knowing, authentic life is grounded in the present. Wherever you go, there you are!

Many people experience spiritual life as simply honoring the beauty found in everyday life. A fifty-year-old student of mine, who is a former runway model and now an interior designer, told me this story of her spiritual renewal:

I took great pride in being able to do forty different things at the same time. I actually trained myself to live my life so that I could scatter myself emotionally and mentally. I would lose things constantly; I was living in the future and couldn't find things like my car keys because they were in the present! I realized that the more efficient I became at this, the less healthy my body felt. Spiritually, I was robbing myself of the simplest pleasures of the present moment that give life true meaning. The meditation sanctuary practice brought me back to the present and gave me the energy to renew my spiritual life and breathe health back into my body.

MEDITATION AS A SACRED PLACE

Your meditation sanctuary connects you with your spirit. It is a place of self-honor and reverence. It is your truth forum; you can ask questions and get answers there. It is a beautiful and loving internal spiritscape. When you first begin to visit your meditation sanctuary, you may have difficulty locating it; you might not feel that you are at the right place. Do not worry, because your sanctuary is a location that does exist, even if you have never frequented its inner site. Simply close your eyes and rest your attention centrally inside your head, and then use your creative imagination to design an interior spiritscape to your liking — an inner comfort zone.

Begin your centering meditation with deep breathing, which helps busy frontal-brain analyzers quiet down. Then move back into your meditation sanctuary by visualizing yourself diving into a river and swimming underwater until you reach a colorful space. When you see a solid color above you from underwater, you'll know you have reached your sanctuary. Then surface and move to a comfortable lounge chair, which conforms to your body. It is from this vantage point that you will observe your body and healing energy. Call your spirit into your sanctuary and greet yourself. Say the affirmation "I am a spirit grounded in my body."

Here is another way to approach your meditation sanctuary: Fill the space with pleasant light and hang banners of beautiful material. Visualize the space as being the perfect size for you, with pillows to sit on, cozy and comfortable. Greet yourself when you enter, saying, *"namaste,"* which is an Eastern greeting of the inner spirit. Set a mood of reverence, respect, and love. Say the affirmation "I am present now in my meditation sanctuary."

The following story is from a current student of Intuition Medicine who is a book designer and poet. An extremely introverted person, she had a difficult time working in a publishing company where everyone was extroverted; this made her anxious and produced feelings of being emotionally crowded, which contributed to her sense of being less creative than her coworkers. She adopted various "hiding" habits in order to feel calm and alone or to ignore her feelings of low self-esteem.

It wasn't until I learned about creating my own sanctuary — a sacred space free of any other people's energy — that I began to experience the reality that I had a safe place to go. Not only that, but I understood that having this safe space was a God-given right. I had used so many strategies in the past to find freedom from the intrusion of others (smoking, drugs, physically hiding, going for long drives alone in the car). Just knowing that I have an inner sanctuary has given me a very serene feeling. It has taken away the anxiety that used to make me want to run and hide from people. Best of all, I can do this while I am surrounded by people.

Images for Your Meditation Sanctuary

People of all ages seek peace and tranquility and need an inner sanctum of healing. I was moved by the writing of a thirteen-year-old who is a teaching assistant in our children's meditation group. In her seventh-grade class, her teacher asked students to write their goals for the year; the last goal on her list is excerpted below. One of the terms used for meditation sanctuary in the children's class is dream place.

One of my goals is to be in my dream place every day. It exists in my mind and is connected to gardens and nature of all kinds. This place is a whole world of my own. No one can decide what my dream place is about except me! It contains flower gardens, still, calm lakes, glittering joy, and pieces of memory from my childhood. A place to rest and be in absolute peace, to ponder on things that are of great importance to me. It is not reality, and what a relief it is to be there.

Right now, visualize some of the following images in your meditation sanctuary location and notice how your mood and perception shift. Focus on the feeling that floods your body when you imagine each of these images.

- A favorite spot in nature
- The top of a mountain
- A light-filled room

- A quiet cave

- A place with a view of the cosmos

- A beautifully decorated room

- A musical amphitheatre

- Feelings of expansiveness

- A big, soft cushion

- A womb of light

- A peaceful garden

DEVELOPING THE THREE FORMS OF CLAIRVOYANCE

With our physical sensory systems, we cannot perceive reality, but can only gain some information about reality. We settle for a set of consistency relationships.[44]

— William Tiller

As you begin to work with the grounding and meditation sanctuary practice, you will naturally develop clairvoyance. Using visualization in your meditations expands all your intuitive skills, notably enhancing clairvoyance. My ability to see energy has been acute for as long as I can recall, so I assumed that everyone "saw" the world with both ocular vision and clairvoyant sight. In my early twenties, I experienced a brief loss of my clairvoyant sight. The world was suddenly flat, not holographic; one-dimensional, not multidimensional; static, not vital. Even my refrigerator lost its gray auric shimmer! When I explained my dilemma to others, most people did not know what I was referring to when I said I could no longer see the "pulse and light" around them.

From years of studying intuitive perception, I have formulated a theory on the development and enhancement of clairvoyance. I observe three aspects of clairvoyant perception, which I refer to as spontaneous clairvoyance, mind's-eye clairvoyance, and intentional clairvoyance. For most people, spontaneous clairvoyance has been forgotten, disconnected, or isolated from their other five senses. Spontaneous clairvoyance is what most people refer to when talking about clairvoyant vision — constant seeing of auras, subtle energy, and so forth — thus often equating it with ocular vision. Most people want to develop spontaneous clairvoyance in intuitive training, as it mirrors the familiar eyesight sense perception; people tend to prefer familiar territory when developing this intuitive sense. However, in the Intuition Medicine model, mind's-eye clairvoyance and intentional clairvoyance are taught in order to stimulate the memory of spontaneous clairvoyance, energetically connect the circuits, and holistically reintegrate and retrain spontaneous clairvoyance to work as autonomically as the other human senses.

Mind's-eye clairvoyance involves receiving a mental image of information, which is seen in one's "mind's eye." This is similar to the process of memory recall; for example, when someone asks you to describe your toothbrush, you would see a memory-image of your toothbrush in your mind's eye or your meditation sanctuary. From that hypothalamus location, you would retrieve the imagery information needed to describe the toothbrush. This process works when you focus inward and your attention is held in the visual receiving area of your brain — the place we are calling the meditation sanctuary or intuitive center. In the realm of intuition, when you look at a person's energy and receive an impression in your meditation sanctuary, this is mind's-eye clairvoyance.

Intentional clairvoyance utilizes a blueprint, template, or other postulated energy mock-up as a holding space for your intentional imagery. This technique assists you in reintegrating spontaneous clairvoyance. To work with this method, you place and hold the intentional energy configuration of something you are scanning — your third chakra, for example, or another person's aura — outside your aura. As you perceive the energy of what you are scanning, this energy-information then registers in your meditation sanctuary.

For example, in our Intuition Medicine training program, we ask a client's permission to do energy work, and then we ask the client to "sign in" by saying his or her name — this saying out loud of one's name has an interesting present-time grounding effect that makes a person's energy easier to sense. We then use psychometry to scan the client's energy field, either doing the psychometric scan directly over the body or visualizing a blueprint of the person's body and energy systems as a technique to intuitively perceive the energy-information. The energy-information registers within the meditation sanctuary — the same location where you saw the image of your toothbrush in the example above. This happens in much the same way that a camera captures an image via light from outside itself and imprints it on the light-sensitive film inside. Your sixth chakra is the lens of the human camera, and the hypothalamus area (or meditation sanctuary) is the light-sensitive film. The translation of the impression you receive into words is part of the ongoing development of your intuitive language.

Spontaneous clairvoyance means seeing energy fields with your eyes open, including perceiving fields of energy directly in or around a life form. We are able to visually see things because our eyes (ocular vision) collect — and our brain decodes — information carried by photons (light waves) as they bounce off the objects being viewed. My theory is that our ocular vision and brain have de-evolved to primarily recognize denser physical matter. Spontaneous clairvoyance is diminished by what appears to be energy "calcification" of the intuitive function of the hypothalamus and the pineal and pituitary glands, as well as by limiting or suppressing the function of the brain in decoding subtle energy fields. In some people, the hardwiring for subtle energy perception is intact, and in others, this function needs to be rewired. In other words, some people naturally observe people's energetic fields along with their physical appearance. For those who do not, rewiring of spontaneous clairvoyance often occurs during the Intuition Medicine practice.

Spontaneous clairvoyance is similar to mind's-eye clairvoyance, but the action of spontaneous clairvoyance is autonomic rather than being a guided imagery process. Spontaneous clairvoyance occurs most often when you are not thinking about it. At first, it may occur quickly as a flash of color, light, symbol, or pattern, which then disappears. With practice and through trusting your intuitive sight, spontaneous clairvoyance becomes stronger and occurs more often, and the energy perception remains visible for longer periods of time. This perception, followed by trust, is one way to reconnect the energetics of the bioelectric wiring that connects our biological and energetic anatomy. The more often you repeat this process, the stronger the signals become, until your "wiring" sustains a hard connection.

Intentional clairvoyance, mind's-eye clairvoyance, and spontaneous clairvoyance are all valid operational modes of clairvoyance. Equally accurate information can be received from each level of clairvoyance, and many intuitive people use all three modes interchangeably. The location of the reception distinguishes these three types of clairvoyance from one another. The more you practice intentional clairvoyance, the stronger your mind's-eye clairvoyance wiring becomes, and the more likely you are to experience spontaneous clairvoyance. Most people find that intentional clairvoyance and mind's-eye clairvoyance work well with the model of Intuition Medicine. A bonus is that, with practice, mind's-eye clairvoyance occurs naturally; for many, it becomes the daily-life, quick intuitive sense.

Now you have a framework for how I understand the aspects of clairvoyance. I have based the Intuition Medicine program on this understanding, training students in formulated learning stages that emphasize practice and repetition. This approach develops a sustained clairvoyant sense. Each practitioner has a different personal timetable for their energetic rewiring or reinstatement of the three modes of clairvoyance.

Reflections and Journaling

Take a few minutes to reflect on the feeling of your meditation sanctuary by reading the lists and questions on the following page and writing about your insights. Please note that there are no absolutes within the study of the human energy field; you will find that some entries overlap or are the same as entries on other chapters' lists. When cross-referencing your journal lists, you may find repetitive or similar entries; this indicates a theme or lesson for you to pay attention to in managing your energy. Use personal experience and discernment in your assessment of all the entries.

Journaling

Look at the following lists. Add to these "In the Present" and "Out of the Present" lists from your experience, then compare the two lists. Write about your insights and feelings in your Intuition Medicine journal.

HOW IT FEELS TO BE...	
IN THE PRESENT	**OUT OF THE PRESENT**
Forehead and face are relaxed	Frazzled, worried, angry, or impatient
Exterior stimulation is in the background	Looping thoughts
Thoughts and words flow without effort	Messing up tasks; needing to repeat tasks
Feelings of trust and compassion	Finding simple activities tedious
Quiet state of mind; no worries	A tendency toward accidents
100 percent focused on the task at hand	Being forgetful or absent-minded
Calm, safe, and feeling infinite potential	Misplacing or losing items easily
Very aware, receptive, and relaxed	Feeling alone or abandoned
Living with inner peace and tranquility	Stuck in analytical mode
Noticing details: All six senses are recording	Obsessing about inconsequential things
Able to feel the location of thought processes	Closed-down heart
Simultaneously in both the inner and outer worlds	Loss of compassion for self or others
Hearing one's inner voice/intuition clearly	Fearful, judgmental, blaming, or critical
Feeling Spirit occupying one's body; not being alone	Loss of objectivity and compassion
Feeling "accompanied" and loved	Tentative or doubtful
	Mentally continuing conversations with others; nonstop head-talk
	Frontal-lobe constriction or headache
	Holding tension in one's brow and face
	Experiencing a cacophony of internal voices

IN THE PRESENT	OUT OF THE PRESENT
Feeling calmness and balance in one's body	A busy feeling inside one's head
A feeling of coming home to one's self	Oblivious to personal needs
A positive/objective response to thoughts and feelings (yours and others')	More into the past or future than the present
Life feels positive	A negative/subjective response to thoughts and feelings (yours and others')
Acceptance of grace in life	Random chaos rather than synchronicity
Confident; no doubts	Life feeling like a struggle rather than a flow
A trusting acceptance of what is	A feeling of buzzing in one's head
A deep feeling of stillness and contentment	Fear and anxiety about the future
A trust that everything is as it should be	Dwelling on past scenarios
Awareness of the larger self and the world	Feelings of having no choice
Clear, immediate, connected external experiences	Thinking about something other than the present activity
Ability to let go of preconceived ideas	Feeling invisible to others
A knowing, innate wisdom	Overanalyzing information
A sense of inner intelligence and caring	Clear ocular vision becoming cloudy
An innate sense of direction and truth	Emotions masking the truth
Sensing universal connection and guiding power	Feeling "forward" and in front of yourself
A sense of lucidity and vastness	Having nagging fears about future possibilities
Feeling responsive to the world without worry, fear, fretting, or anxiety	Internal dialogues about other people's issues
Connection with a nonlinear, knowing state	Easily losing patience
Feelings of compassionate neutrality	Being overly emotional
Calm and keenly aware of surroundings	

Reflections

Think about the symptoms that tell you when you are in your meditation sanctuary and those that tell you when you are not. How can you quickly know when you are in or out of your meditation sanctuary? You know that you are in your meditation sanctuary when you have a wider, objective view of the world and therefore take things less personally, and also when you can experience a highly emotional event while being fully present. You know that you are not in your meditation sanctuary when thoughts repetitively run through your mind, you are judgmental about yourself and others, and you obsess about past events.

Think about times in your life when you have been in your meditation sanctuary and have experienced being present. What was happening to you? Think about times in your life when you have not been in the present. What activities were you engaged in while in the present and out of the present? Who were you with, or were you alone? What were you doing or thinking?

Using these sensations as your intuition language, you can become more aware of how you subtly interact with others and the world around you. Next time you notice any of your symptoms of being in the present, stop and notice the immediate interaction, thoughts, or situation you are involved in. These symptoms are reminders that your intuitive energy information processing is active. Learn to notice and act on these subtle messages, and you will reap the benefit of a centered focus every day.

More Reflections and Journaling

Take some time to reflect on how you operate in the world in relation to the intuitive concept of living in the present. Make notes in your journal about which side of the following list contains the most descriptions of your experiences — or add to these lists from your own experiences.

ACTIVITIES AND THINGS THAT...

ENHANCE LIVING IN THE PRESENT	WEAKEN LIVING IN THE PRESENT
Meditation	Angry or ungrounded people
Making a conscious effort to be present	Dominance or control
Relaxing your facial muscles	Trying too hard; operating with effort
Smiling intentionally	Engaging in power struggles
Practicing trust and compassion	Fear and anxiety
Aromatherapy; certain smells	Frantic business
Breathing deeply	Too much external stimulation
Eating with enjoyment	Anticipation; a future-oriented attitude
Feelings of stillness; slowing down	Being ungrounded
Spirit-to-spirit greeting	Practicing perfection; acting from one's inner critic
Listening, journaling	Replaying past events excessively
Focused creative endeavors	Obsessively needing to figure things out
Looking at people with love and respect	Lack of exercise
Listening to people with compassion	Undereating
Giving/receiving a massage	Abusive use of alcohol or drugs
Living in integrity	Crowds and noise
Being in nature	Spending time with people who are out of integrity
Practicing nonattachment to outcomes	Stressing and hurrying
Eating good chocolate slowly	Dependence on linear, analytical reason
Affirming that your analytical mind is on vacation	Victim consciousness
Playing with children	Deadlines and unexpected difficulties
	Personal anger or disappointment

Reflections

Think about the activities in the foregoing lists and answer these questions:

- Which specific events or people cause you to feel out of your meditation sanctuary?

- Which events or people help you feel in your meditation sanctuary and in the present?

- Why do these events and people affect you in this way?

Journaling

Take a moment to think about these things and write about them in your journal. These reflective questions will help you become aware of how you experience your meditation sanctuary and the present moment.

I hope that this chapter on the meditation sanctuary has given you a new, better, or possibly larger perspective on reality. I hope that it has enhanced your ability to participate in the world with more vital energy, as a force for the greater good, empowered with inner knowledge and practical intuition tools.

Go to the next chapter, "The Meditation Sanctuary Practice," when you feel ready to put the perspectives and intuitions you received from this chapter into your living awareness of yourself, others, and your participation in the world.

Chapter 7

THE MEDITATION SANCTUARY PRACTICE

One's destination is never a place, but rather a new way of looking at things.

— Henry Miller

After reading the previous chapter, you may feel ready to practice the perception-enhancing tool of the meditation sanctuary. I suggest that you read this chapter completely, then choose whichever mode appeals to you most and practice that one — a good way to use your intuition for making a choice!

This chapter includes six sections, covering the contemplative, observational, daily-living, experimental, affirmation-setting, and introspective practices of staying present in your meditation sanctuary. You might experiment with using one of these modes of practice for a few days — for example, the daily awareness practice — then focusing on the contemplative meditations for the next few days. Try to practice with all the modes in this chapter before you integrate the other meditation practices that follow in the book, as I believe that this area of intuitive awareness is critical in mastering the more subtle skills of diagnosis and energy healing that are presented later.

Contemplative Meditations

These two meditation sanctuary meditations enable you to find, feel, and know the location of your intuitive center of perception. You may need practiced repetition to fully sustain your ability to be present in the meditation sanctuary, both in a contemplative meditation and in daily-awareness practice. The first meditation is designed to locate you in your meditation sanctuary; it is a good one to practice when you choose to bring yourself to a quiet state of mind. The second meditation presents a method of intuitive inquiry that you may use for introspection, diagnosis, or self-healing. In intuitive inquiry, it is a good habit to trust your first insight — the one that comes in a flash or a blink. The second, third, and later pieces of information probably come from your analytical mind, which performs the rote function of relating stored analytical responses.

You may choose to do the two meditations one after the other or to do each alone. Your intuition will be strengthened when you take a few minutes after each meditation to reflect on your experiences. In order to go deeper into observational learning, I suggest that you answer the post-meditation questions after each of the meditations, then write notes on your personal insights in your journal.

Meditation Sanctuary

- Find a comfortable, quiet place to meditate. Close your eyes and begin to breathe slowly, inhaling through your nose and exhaling through your mouth. Breathe with the intention of slowing down and relaxing. Focus on listening to the sound of your breath. Do this for about a minute, then let your breathing return to a natural rhythm.

- Come into communication with yourself by bringing your attention into your head and resting it in the area of your hypothalamus gland — your meditation sanctuary. (See the Meditation Sanctuary illustration on page 75.) Greet yourself. Hear, sense, and feel the presence of your inner voice. Mentally say hello to yourself to establish a ritual coming into sacred space.

- Within your meditation sanctuary, design a sacred space. Use your creative imagination and decorate the interior with colors, sounds, smells, and emotions. This is your sacred personal space; you can reside in your sanctuary at peace with yourself, with no other people or distractions. When needed, clean out any lingering distractions by either grounding off or acknowledging the energy, then asking the energy to leave; sometimes a gentle push helps. Be in your sacred space and feel the quiet experience. Be in a no-thought place. Hold that feeling and energy for a quiet minute.

- With your attention in your meditation sanctuary, visualize the energy of your spiritual self as a color, symbol, or knowing; experience the energy of yourself as spirit. Greet and embrace your spirit. Visualize a current of your spiritual energy moving from the center of your meditation sanctuary down through your body and into the center of the earth. Visualize anchoring your spirit through your body into Mother Earth. See and feel your spirit coming more fully into your body. Breathe deeply and relax. Hold that feeling of sacred spirit for a minute.

Meditation Sanctuary and Intuitive Inquiry

- Find a comfortable, quiet place to meditate. Close your eyes and begin to breathe slowly, inhaling through your nose and exhaling through your mouth. Breathe with the intention of slowing down and relaxing. Focus on listening to the sound of your breath. Do this for about a minute, then let your breathing return to a natural rhythm.

- Be present in your meditation sanctuary. Greet yourself and ground your spirit through your body into Mother Earth. Hold that feeling for a minute.

- Greet yourself again and focus on listening to the sound and feeling of your inner voice. Continue to greet yourself with the intention of experiencing your spirit residing in the center of your head. Repeat until you are centered in this place of the Now.

- For diagnosis or self-healing inquiry, sit quietly, focused within yourself, in a relaxed place of receiving. The information is already present and available to you. Cultivate a quiet watching and inner-listening posture in order to receive the information.

- Clearly formulate a question and, with your inner voice, intuitively state that question. Sit quietly, watch, wait, and be present. Often the answer comes very quickly, so you must be alert and trust the *first* insight you receive.

- You may receive answers via knowing, psychometry, clairvoyance, clairaudience, telepathy, clairsentience, or a combination of your intuitive abilities.

- If you wonder whether you have mentally created the answer, you probably have! When you receive an accurate reply to your inquiry, you will experience a sense of knowing.

- After you receive a response to each inquiry, make a closure with that question before you move on to another inquiry. Remember to write all your insights in your journal.

Observational Practice: Journaling

If you wish, write notes and reflections in your journal in response to the following questions. It is always more fruitful to do this practice immediately following one or both of the meditation sanctuary meditations.

Post-Meditation Questions

1. What did you learn about your meditation sanctuary as a location?

2. Note how you received your information when you asked questions from your meditation sanctuary. Was it through images, sounds, words, feeling, symbols, colors, or knowing?

3. How did you sense when you were present in your meditation sanctuary during meditation?

4. How do you sense when you are present in your meditation sanctuary while out in the world?

5. Is perceiving from your meditation sanctuary a familiar feeling?

6. How do you know or experience the Now?

7. Write affirmations inspired by your practice of being present in the Now.

Daily-Living Tips

- Often during the day, pause and affirm being present in your meditation sanctuary.

- Perceive others as spiritual and physical beings. Practice greeting others spirit-to-spirit.

- Practice awareness of activities, locations, and people that tend to move you out of the integrity of your meditation sanctuary.

- Practice awareness of activities, locations, and people that enhance your ability to be present in the Now.

Experiments: Try This!

- Try this to stimulate and develop inner seeing and clairvoyance. Sit in a dark room. Focus your attention in your meditation sanctuary and keep your eyes open; remain awake and conscious. You will eventually begin to see light although there is no outer source of light. This is a good practice for stimulating clairvoyance. (see "Developing the Three Forms of Clairvoyance" on page 89 of chapter 6.)

- Practice greeting others spirit-to-spirit. After you say a greeting of *physical recognition* to a person in whatever language you speak — hello, *aloha, bonjour, ciao, jambo, néih hóu, salam* — give an inner-voice greeting of *spiritual recognition* to the person.

As a note of interest, some people practice this type of greeting as part of their culture. The formal greeting of spiritual and physical recognition in Hindu tradition, *namaste*, is accomplished by raising one's hands, clasped together in a prayerlike gesture, to one's forehead or sixth chakra. *namaste* translates as "The light within me honors the light within you."

Affirmations: Repeat Often

- I am happy, not perfect.

- I am centered in the middle of chaos.

- I live in my body and am emotionally grounded.

- I practice compassion and objectivity.

- I respond to life's unfolding treasures.

- I enjoy the present moment.

- I am in the world, connecting deeply with her natural flow and beauty.

- In every moment, I am a prosperous expression of my creative, spiritual self.

Trust

Grow and expand your intuition and creativity. Be in a loving relationship with yourself. Practice detachment from currently held beliefs and assumptions, allowing higher wisdom to enter and give you a vision of wholeness. Meditate and integrate.

Chapter 8

LIFE-FORCE AND EARTH ENERGY: YOUR PERSONAL HEALING ENERGY

At the heart of each of us, whatever our imperfections, there exists a silent pulse of perfect rhythm, a complex of wave forms and resonances, which is absolutely individual and unique, and yet which connects us to everything in the universe.

— George Leonard

Life-force and earth energy naturally circulates through your body, organs, tissues, and cells, clearing out old negative energy and replenishing you with new, vibrant energy — this combination is an inner pharmacopeia of natural medicine. Your personal meditation practice locates, amplifies, and directs this energy, creating a profound healing effect on your body, mind and spirit. At times this natural inducer of health is diminished and we need to find ways to revive our well-being. In what follows, you will learn about powerful life-enhancing tools for bringing balance and energy to your life.

LIFE AS ENERGY AND MEDICINE

Many sciences have studied the origins of life in order to define the life force. Quantum biology is the study of invisible matter and interrelates light, life force, and human biology. The superstring theory in physics describes the invisible force of life as elementary particles of matter that are vibrations of infinitesimally small strands, called superstrings.[1] This theory postulates that all particles of matter and light are manifestations of these particles. Like the strings of a guitar that vibrate together, they produce a unified harmony that fills nature.[2]

The harmony and health of life-force energy is dependent on many factors, one of which is that living things depend on essential coherence in order to function, adapt, evolve, and thrive. Healthy living systems are organized in patterns; the energy field characteristic of a living system is a basic property of life.[3] In the science of Intuition Medicine, the life force is defined as the coherent, patterned, and essential vivifying energy generated with your first breath at birth and extinguished with your last dying breath — it is the sustenance of life and the pulse of health. Normal light is incoherent light, vibrating in random directions and phases over a wide range of frequencies. In contrast, coherent light vibrates in phase in one direction and usually at a single frequency, as in a monochromatic laser. Coherent light interacts with matter very strongly, and that is when remarkable things can happen. Electroencephalogram (EEG) studies indicate that increased coherence in the functioning of the human brain is a key feature of meditation practice.[4]

Chinese and ayurvedic medicine recognize subtle energy meridian networks in the human anatomy that integrate the physical body with the spiritual body. These networks, called *nadis*, are measured as octaves of the electromagnetic spectrum that parallel the nervous system. This subtle nadi vibration is described as "threads of energy."[5] Might these threads correlate with what physicists call superstrings?

The definition of life energy is explored by many others, with complementary parallels to my definition. For the purposes of our study, life force-energy is your natural inner medicine of healing.

Do you sense when your body needs medicine or something else to feel better? A second-year practitioner of Intuition Medicine, who is a fifty-year-old hospital chaplain diagnosed with hepatitis C, told me of her healing experience:

The most telling and beautiful experience I've ever had was when the power of combined earth energy and life-force energy was revealed to me during a meditation. During this meditation, I directed this healing force to an area of my body: my liver, which needed healing. At that moment, I received the message loud and clear that I was no longer sick. I had a sense of knowing such as I had never known before. I became very emotional, and my tears flowed. My next blood tests revealed that not only were my liver enzymes completely normal, but the virus had disappeared from my blood! While I don't discredit Western medicine, I don't give it full credit for my body returning to health.

LIFE-FORCE VIBRATION

There is only one health, but diseases are many. Likewise there appears to be one fundamental force that heals, although with a myriad of ways of cajoling it into action.[6]

— Robert Becker

I theorize that your life force is your personal vivifying harmonic vibration — the life-force energy responsible for your experience of who you are. Your health and well-being are dependent on the vital presence of this energy. Some biologists speak of an "inherent vitality" that is strong at birth and fades out during life; the more rapidly it is consumed, the sooner one ages and dies. In the following passage, physiologist and psychologist Valerie Hunt comments on her experience with individual energy signatures (I have included my analogous terms in brackets).

My research shows that the human energy fields display a continuum. The extremely low frequencies [earth energy] are directly involved in life's biological processes. The extremely high-frequency [life-force] patterns ally with the mind-field and awareness. The general pattern of extremely

low frequencies is similar for all people, while the extremely high fre-
quency reveals a personal signature of emotional patterning for each
person.

To understand the individual emotional signatures, the steady state to
which one returns, requires a search in the high-frequency patterns of
people. Lower vibrations exist with material reality, higher ones with mys-
tical reality, and a full vibration spectrum [combined life-force and earth
energy] with expanded reality.[7]

Your life-force energy is your personal vibration signature. It is unique
to you in the universe. Each brain and body is a little different from every
other brain and body in the world. Among the billions of fingerprints
around the world, even among identical twins, no two identical fingerprints have been found.[8] Like an energy fingerprint, your life force identifies you as an individual being, distinct from all other beings and
energies. In his unified theory of the universe, physicist William Tiller
draws an analogy between the information-receiving capacities of the television and those of the human body; this is similar to my description of
the personal signature vibration. What Tiller calls the God-given frequency is similar to what I call the life-force energy.

Let us contrast a similar analogy for people by assuming that each indi-
vidual has a God-given frequency which is the carrier wave of the in-
dividual (it is unchanging). The evolution of this individual is
characterized by their growth in consciousness, or the fulfilling of the infor-
mation capacity inherent in his/her frequency.[9]

Life-force energy can be heard as a sound (a human sonic frequency)
by some clairaudient people. If you feel better when listening to certain
sounds and music and are adversely affected by others, you can use sound
as a healing tool. The Bio-Acoustics healing method uses a unique
approach to sound signature vibrations, based on the discovery of individual human sonic frequencies. Experimentation with audiotapes con-
taining recordings of sonic frequencies led to the discovery that the

sounds had healing effects on listeners, but only when the listeners heard their own unique note or frequency. Furthermore, when a frequency was missing from a person's energy field, various healing effects occurred upon listening to that missing note or sound frequency.[10]

An Intuition Medicine practitioner had a powerful experience of her own life force:

> *After hearing about the personal life-force energy, I realize I have experienced my personal life-force energy but didn't call it such. During my life-force meditation, I affirmed seeing my life-force symbol. The first thing that came to my mind was a picture of a spark of Divine energy, and it wasn't just a concept; I felt the Divine spark. I was in awe of it, and the most awesome thing I felt was that the Divine spark was me! The Divine and I are the same, and there is no separation! I heard a voice saying, over and over again, "There is no separation; you are the same!" I experienced my personal life-force energy as the Divine's unique expression through me. I feel as if I am as valuable as the most holy person who has ever walked the earth, and that is true for every person.*

Life-Force Energy Cross-References

Many traditions and philosophies have concepts comparable to that of the life force:

Chinese: *chi*

Hindu: *prana*

Sufi: *baraka*

Algonquin Indians: *manitu*

African Masai: *ngai*

Paracelsus: *archaeus* or *liquor vitae*

Aristotle: formative cause

Hippocrates: *vis medicatrix naturae*

Goethe: *gestaltung*
J.B. Rhine: Psi faculty
Eeman: X-Force
Bergson: *élan vital*
Theosophists: biomagnetism
Vitalists: life force
Medieval alchemy: vital fluid or divine water
van Helmont: *magnale magnum*
Fludd: *spiritus*
Galvani: life force
Mesmer: animal magnetism
Brunler: dielectric radiation or bio-cosmic energy
Reichenbach: odic force
Jung: synchronicity
Maslow: synergy
Reich: orgone

Body of Light-Force

Clear is the pathway to he who has wisdom.
Open the door to the kingdom of light.[11]

— Thoth

Quantum physics and the study of the subatomic world take on mystical meaning when we view the world through the principle of quantum calculations. These show that we and our universe live and breathe in what amounts to a sea of motion — a quantum sea of light.[12] The photoreceptors in the retina of the human eye — the flavin molecules — are also found in virtually every tissue of the body.[13] Our human biology reacts to light in a healing manner called photo-repair. In the laboratory, biologists have exposed a cell to enough ultraviolet light to destroy 99 percent of the cell, including its DNA. Then, by illuminating the same cells with the same wavelength of light of a very weak intensity, they have been able to almost entirely repair the damage in a single day. Recent research and the development of subtle-light measurement instruments indicates that there is light in the body that is responsible for photo-repair.[14] In 1970, theoretical biophysicist Fritz-Albert Popp discovered that light in the body may hold the key to health and illness. He used his "light machine" to measure biophoton emissions as a gauge for measuring health and regeneration. He discovered that all living things emit a permanent current of photons (particles of light) and that the current is related to an organism's position on the evolutionary scale.

In another experiment, light was shone on living cells; the cells took in this light and, after a certain delay, shone intensely — a process called delayed luminescence. The living system apparently had to maintain a delicate equilibrium of light (10 photons per square centimeter per second, at a wavelength of 200 to 800 nanometers), and when it was bombarded with too much light, it would reject the excess.[15] It is of interest to note that when you intentionally direct life-force energy into an area of the human body and the area reaches saturation, no more energy will be accepted; by placing your hands at that area, you can psychometrically feel the overflow energy pushing out.

If all your cells are healthy — filled to capacity with life force — you cannot be sick. According to Len Saputo, MD, cellular malfunction is the root cause of all disease.[16] In further investigation of the correlation between light and life, consider the fact that human DNA vibrates at 52 to 78 gigahertz (GHz) — and that sunlight also bathes the earth at 52 to 78 GHz.[17]

Low-level light therapy, first proposed by Albert Einstein in 1917, is finding a place in contemporary sports medicine. In February 2004, an article in the *Washington Post* described the use of photo-repair technology to successfully treat injured athletes:

> *The New England Patriots won Super Bowl XXXVIII with some help from a little-known form of laser technology that could change the way athletic injuries and chronic pain are treated.*[18]

The article went on to report that, during the week preceding the Super Bowl, more than ten Patriot players were treated with cold laser therapy for tendon and muscle injuries. The laser expedited healing of some players' soreness and pain. The team nurse/physical therapist said that the improved recoveries were not a coincidence: for example, the treatment was used on one player's flared-up sciatic nerve, and he experienced relief soon after treatment.

The Circle of Light

Intuition is the language of light through which men and God intercommunicate.[19]

— Walter Russell

All living things depend on light for life. Imagine yourself filled with light. Now imagine yourself filled with darkness. For most sentient beings, a lengthy absence of light brings on despair and ultimately leads to death. Physicists have long considered the entire physical world to consist of various manifestations of light. Under special circumstances, light and matter can interchange; in fact, matter is sometimes referred to as frozen light.[20] Humans are photosynthetic — we use light as food by absorbing light through solar energy cells that are all over the skin and inside the body. In the absence of light, humans suffer from what some researchers refer to as malillumination.[21] The biblical admonition "Do not hide your light under a basket"[22] takes on new meaning when we think of light as life force. I theorize that your life-force energy is the light of your spirit and the inner medicine of health and well-being. Through the practice of life-force meditation heliotherapy (medical therapy involving exposure to sunlight), healing occurs and feelings of well-being are increased.

All living things constantly emit light and vibration. Your life-force energy is always present in your body, pulsing with the rhythm of life. The quantity and quality of this pulsation vary with your state of health and mind and your interaction with other energies. *Your light and vibration are your life-force energy*, and this energy holds the keys to health and illness. Your light vibration holds information, and information is the currency of health.

Read the following list and see if these feelings are familiar to you.

How Life-Force Energy Feels

- Happy, very alive

- A light, refreshing tingle

- A diamondlike glow

- A soothing pulse, like a heartbeat

- Like a vibrating tuning fork

- Integrated vitality emanating from within

FEET ON THE EARTH

With your feet on the ground, you may feel the pulse of the earth. With your ear to the ground, you may hear the heartbeat of Mother Earth. The second major source of energy that moves throughout your body is the earth's electromagnetic field, acted upon and modified by the life-force field within your body.

Mystics' brainwaves, regenerative healing, and the pulse of the earth resonate within a few cycles per second of one another, suggesting a deep interconnectedness of spirit, body, and earth. The earth behaves like an enormous electric circuit, pulsing electromagnetic waves. The earth's background base frequency, or "heartbeat," is 7.83 cycles per second and is called the Schumann Resonance.

In the laboratory, the brain waves of mystics who were channeling universal information have been recorded at 7.8 cycles per second. The micro-motion of a healthy human body fluctuates at about 6.8 to 7.8 cycles per second. These correlations suggest that, in deep meditation, a constant resonant tuning and healing occurs between a meditator and the earth.[23]

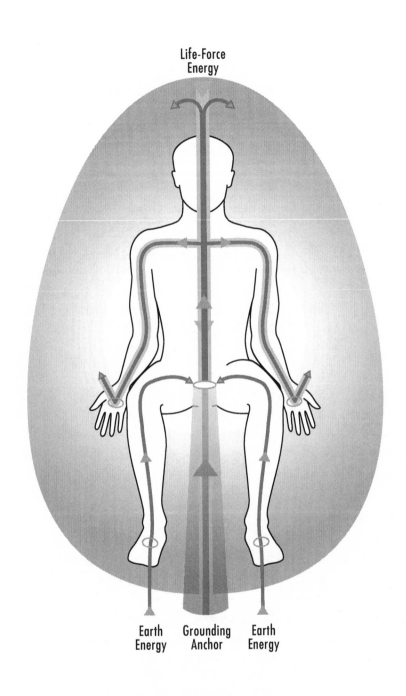

Life-Force
Energy

Earth   Grounding   Earth
Energy   Anchor   Energy

GROUNDING, LIFE-FORCE ENERGY, AND EARTH ENERGY

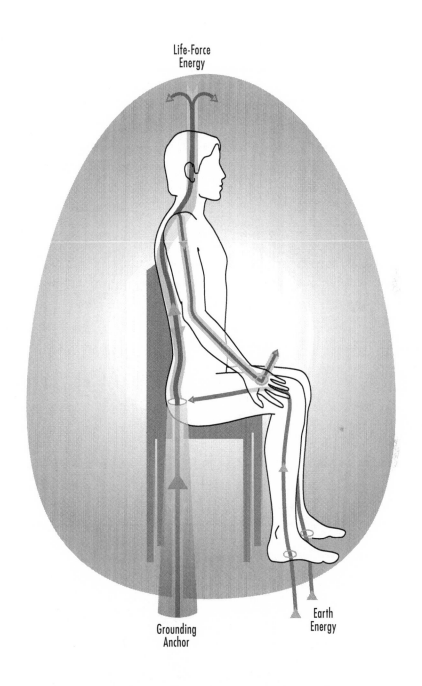

Life-Force
Energy

Grounding
Anchor

Earth
Energy

SIDE VIEW: GROUNDING, LIFE-FORCE ENERGY, AND EARTH ENERGY

The earth is constantly bathing all living things in her natural frequency, her rhythmic pulsation — the brain wave of the earth. Most of us are exposed to a wide range of artificial electromagnetic signals that overwhelm this natural, beneficial pulse of the earth. The characteristics of the earth's energy field (electromagnetic and gravitational) vary with location. Living organisms are entrained by the local energy fields where they live, possibly experiencing beneficial as well as detrimental effects. If you choose to live in a certain country, city, or neighborhood because it "feels" good, you may be clairsentiently feeling the geographic network of the earth's energy field, called ley lines, which may be Mother Earth's acupuncture meridians.[24]

Your body is a transducer of earth energy. You are capable of generating an amplified earth-energy pulse through yourself for regeneration and vitality and as a source of natural medicine for body, mind, and spirit. Living in a technological world, you need an extra dose of natural electromagnetic energy to offset high-tech electrical energy for a constant state of health.

Medical acupuncture is demonstrating a health connection between earth energy and the body. A brochure describing the health benefits of Chinese medicine states the following:

> *The natural magnetic field of the earth is in decline and is presently at its lowest level since humans inhabited the planet. Scientists have come to realize that there is a definitive relationship between the earth's magnetic field and the magnetic properties of our bodies. Any change in this earth-energy field is likely to cause functional disorders in the body.*[25]

All life on earth is dependent on the background magnetic energy of Mother Earth, which cradles living cells in a nurturing and orienting energy environment.[26] Most indigenous cultures revere the power of the earth and her life-giving force, and many religions and mystical traditions have centered on symbolism and worship of Mother Earth.

The human organism maintains its functioning balance through a dynamic information exchange between its various systems and the earth. Information exchange occurs at all levels within the body. Human bodily fluids act as important carriers of bio-information; paramagnetic substances in the blood act like magnetic tape, carrying and delivering information throughout the body.[27]

Kyoichi Nakagawa, MD, director of Tokyo's Isuzu Hospital, has studied the effects of the earth's magnetic field on human health. He finds that many people do not get adequate magnetic-field exposure for optimal function due to the earth's decreasing magnetic field. Dr. Nakagawa describes the common symptoms of this deficiency: stiffness of the shoulders, back, and scruff of the neck; lumbago of uncertain cause; chest pains for no specific reason; habitual headache and heaviness of the head; dizziness and insomnia for uncertain reasons; habitual constipation; and general lassitude. He goes on to state that, by providing a natural magnetic field for the body by contact with the earth, many discomforts may be lessened or vanish completely.[28] If you experience any of these symptoms, work with Intuition Medicine to see if meditation alleviates the maladies. I have included the "Health Issues" chart in appendix 1 as a guide for you in this healing practice.

The practice of earth-energy meditation (see page 132) can provide you with an increased natural magnetic field. It sensitizes your body to recognize the beneficial feeling of the earth's pulse and to notice when your body is operating with a diminished earth pulse.[29]

Love Mother Earth

All you need is love...[30]

— The Beatles

Research done at the Institute of HeartMath revealed a fascinating phenomenon. This work tended to confirm the theory that love is a real healing energy with measurable physiological effects, even at the level of DNA. One experiment involved meditators who were able to produce a coherent love-associated heart pattern. A special coil was hooked up to a tree to create living antennae that would measure the earth's local magnetic field while the meditators generated love-energy. During the moment of love's presence, a coherent series of spectral-frequency harmonics appeared in both the loving meditator and the earth's local magnetic field, as measured by the nearby tree. Measurements were in frequencies up to and including 7.8 Hz. The implications of a resonant energy connection between loving emotions and the planetary magnetic field are profound. We are inextricably interwoven with the life-giving properties of Mother Earth. Earth energy is information, and this energy information sustains and supports our experience of being alive.[31]

Read the following list and note whether you have felt these earth-energy sensations in your body.

How Earth Energy Feels

- Soothing, slow

- Warm and tingly in feet and legs

- Connected

- A warm, ancient, yet ever-new, pulsing river of mud

- Solid, heavy energy

A SYMPHONY OF LIFE AND EARTH

Pick a flower and trouble a star.[32]

— Stanley Krippner

Expanded consciousness encompasses a complete spectrum of vibrations; grounding in the lower frequencies of earth energy combines with great power in the higher frequencies of your life force.[33] Consciousness is understood as the subjective experience of being a human individual with mental activity and a spiritual personality separate from those of other individuals. I postulate that in order to be a fully realized human being — a conscious spirit living in a body — one must experience one's unique individuation before wisdom can be present and before a true appreciation and love of all others can be experienced. Grounding your awareness in everyday reality and in the electromagnetic vibrations of the earth must come first in any attempt to understand mystical problems.[34]

All matter is composed of a matrix of light and magnetism. Intentional meditation on your life force and on earth energy (see the next chapter) will harmonize your spirit and body in a unified field of consciousness so that you can experience a fully realized life. Wisdom, intuition, health, and the knowledge of how to maintain this state of well-being are all present within you as an inherent part of your existence.

The Healing Practice of Life-Force and Earth Energy

Roget's Thesaurus describes the divine spark as "the vital force within living beings."[35] Life-force and earth energy are always present in your system. The quantity and quality of these energies will vary depending on how you are feeling, thinking, and interacting with the world around you, along with many other factors. A healthy energy system allows the life-force and earth energy to flow unrestricted throughout the physical body as well as through the subtle-energy systems of the chakras, aura, and grounding.

As you learn to recognize the resonance of your personal life force and the earth's energy, you will be better able to recognize when either of these energies is lacking. You will also be able to sense whether there are other unhealthy energies within your system. With this awareness, you can choose to vitalize your life-force and earth energy and to direct unhealthy energy out of your personal space. The meditation practice of earth energy and life force upgrades and maintains your spiritual sense of self and your physical health, and it gives you a tool for maintaining this state of health.

You might think of earth energy as your system's cleanser and your life force as the polisher. Earth energy has a natural ability to attract negative or aberrant energy from your space and carry it down and out of your system, following the force of gravity. Your personal life force can then be directed through visualization or intention to fill the space that has been cleared by the earth energy. This is a simple, highly effective practice for maintaining your sense of health and well-being. It is also a practice that you can do at any time, in any place.

Life-Force and Earth-Energy Pathways

Great souls are they who see that spiritual is stronger than material force, that thoughts rule the world.[36]

— Ralph Waldo Emerson

There are many pathways in your body through which various types of healing energy flow and numerous universal force energies. Earth energy and life force follow specific pathways in your body.

Earth energy enters your body through your open feet chakras, located at the soles of your feet. It fills your feet and flows up your legs through channels that connect into your first chakra, then flows back down into the earth. The action of this strong circular pathway of earth energy through the lower part of your body creates a gravity pull that enhances your grounded connection to the earth. Dissonant energy, aberrant feelings, and mirrored emotions within your system are directed to the ground and pulled down into the earth, where they are converted into a neutral resonance. This is a sort of reclamation process; energy is not lost, as the geomagnetic grounding reestablishes the released energy to its original resonant pulse. (See the Grounding Life-Force and Earth Energy illustrations on pages 114–115.)

I often hear comments from my students that they do not want to "pollute" the earth with their negative energy or that one should transform "negative energy" into love before releasing it. I think this is a difficult task for the average person and that the healthiest approach is to simply release the negative energy into the neutral field of the earth. Gaia uses it as fertilizer!

A primary-school teacher who is a first-year Intuition Medicine practitioner had the following comment about grounding negative energy:

I was hesitant at first to send energy that I viewed as "negative" into the earth. A theory I had read somewhere stated that all negative energy should be transformed into love before being released, so as not to release any more negativity into the world. I came to experience that the magnetic force of

the earth acts as a neutralizer. It acts as a giant magnet for all unwanted
energy in my system. With this practice, I now feel more like myself!

Your life force operates within the closed circuit of your personal space, which is bounded by the edge of your aura. Within this closed field of personal energy, the natural directional flow of life force enters your body at your seventh chakra and flows down through your head and neck and along your back through subtle channels on either side of your spine, then into the first chakra at the base of your spine. At the first chakra, the earth energy and life force combine in a gyromagnetic mix, which can be visualized as magnets adhering together and spinning in a circle. That energetic mix travels up the front of your body, moving energy through the seven major chakras along your spine and flows out the top of your head into your aura. When the life force reaches your fifth chakra (at the throat), some of the energy flows across your shoulders, down your arms, into your hand chakras, and out into your aura, where it is distributed throughout your auric field. The life-force energy continues in this flux and flow, automatically continuing this revitalizing distribution process. Your life-force energy is a homecoming — an experience of feeling truly alive. Life force holds your potential — your connection with your personal journey.

An unimpeded flux and flow of this personal energy mix is indicative of a natural state of health and gives you a feeling of well-being. Visualization and intention can help you direct this energy to areas that need healing and cleansing. You can cleanse and heal your physical body, grounding, chakras, and aura with this energy mix. When this current is impeded, your health and well-being are compromised, but personal success can heighten your experience of life force.

Life force is more ethereal and energizing than earth energy, which is powerful in its low frequency and brings a deep sense of quiet. Earth energy has a feeling of richness and thickness, while life force is that spark of Spirit-life that is given to everyone. Both of these energies are necessary for pulling your spirit into your body and keeping it there. It may be easy to call your spirit in, but the duration of its presence in your body is sustained when you practice grounding, life-force, and earth-energy meditations first (see details in chapters 5 and 9).

I developed my system of life-force and earth-energy work from personal healing observations and clinical sessions with thousands of clients. Only later did I discover the similarities between my practice and the research of other healers, scientists, and teachers.

LIFE-FORCE AND EARTH-ENERGY PERSPECTIVES

The sky begins at your feet.[37]

— Hopi chant

A daily dose of life-force and earth-energy meditation (see chapter 9) is essential to feeling good, and it is a remedy when you are feeling out of sorts. The alchemy of these energies brings you the potential of fresh, energized, ready, open, strong, graceful experiences of yourself, grounded with wit and laughter and mixed with wisdom, compassion, and neutrality. This is a highly recommended recipe for a vital life.

A social worker who is a second-year Intuition Medicine practitioner found it life-changing to work with earth energy:

> *Most of my life was spent taking everyone else's energy into my space. I didn't realize that the reason I always felt so stressed out, hyperemotional, and generally bad was that I was feeling everyone's energy except mine. Working with earth energy is always calming. I do an earth-energy bath at least once a day, if not more, to slow myself down and ground off excess charge and other energies. I initially found it difficult to allow myself to connect deeply with earth energy; emotionally, I didn't know how to accept the support it gives me. But, increasingly, I can see and feel how much my physical and emotional bodies really need that earth connection and how beneficial it is.*

You can also visualize or intend to change the proportions of earth energy and life force running through your body. There will be times in your day when you will need the grounding, clearing effects of earth energy, and other times when you will need to increase the energizing, personal vibration of your life force. In terms of calming your nervous system, you may find that meditating with grounding and earth energy is as good as getting a massage or taking a yoga class. The next time you wake up in the middle of the night, try grounding and moving earth energy through your entire body as an antidote to insomnia. When you are hyperactive or anxious during the day, use this practice to quiet yourself. During exercise, you will be more present in your physical body if you include this energy practice. Using earth energy to define your personal space helps you to stay more solidly in your center. As you come to recognize the pulse of these energies, you can manage their combination and direct it where it is most needed.

Earth energy engenders a greater appreciation for Gaia and all things connected with her — manifestations of the spirit-life of the earth. Life force and earth energy are a coming together that inspires awe and enjoyment of life and enlivens you to speak, act, and listen from a place of wisdom. Life force and earth energy combined with grounding in the Now is a potent personal alchemy.

A homemaker and practitioner of Intuition Medicine comments on her experience:

> All my life, I just wanted to feel comfortable and safe in my own body. I searched through people, religion, drugs, gurus, books, healing work, doctors, lovers, and on and on. As I get more grounded and in touch with earth energy and my own life-force energy, I realize that this is the closest I have ever felt to a sort of consistent peace in my own body, and that I can feel this way all day and every day.

Reflections and Journaling

As you integrate the life-force and earth-energy practice into your life and adapt its meditations and intentions for your personal health benefit, it is useful to make time for reflective self-assessments.

Reflection

I provide the following self-reflective questions to give you a mental break and allow you to intuitively feel and energetically internalize the information you have just read.

- Think about your connection to earth energy. Scan your typical week and notice the times when you are around devices such as computers, cell phones, and televisions or in buildings that disconnect you from earth energy.

- Now notice the times during your week when you feel especially close to nature and the earth.

- Take an intuitive guess at the amount of earth energy and life force that are running through your body right now.

LIFE-FORCE AND EARTH-ENERGY IMAGES

You can visualize the healing energy of the life-force and earth energy all day as a continuous flow throughout your body. Any image that works for you is good. Here are some suggestions:

- Light above and earth below

- A waterfall cascading into deep tree roots

- A tree of life

- Being cradled in the arms of Mother Earth

- Sitting on top of a mountain with sunlight pulsing through your body

- Two different notes sounding a harmonious blend

LIFE-FORCE AND EARTH ENERGY: WHEN TO ADD MORE

Energy is like a spice; the right type and amount create a satisfying experience. Look at the lists of activities on the following pages and use them as a recipe for healing yourself.

YOU NEED MORE...	
LIFE FORCE	**EARTH ENERGY**
When you feel lethargic or sluggish	When you feel ungrounded or clumsy
To relieve depression or irritability	When your mind feels foggy
To enhance creative expression	To clear sadness
In social situations	When working near electronic equipment
To speak or assert yourself during meetings	In times of anxiety or stress
To speed recovery from a cold, flu, or other illness	When fighting off a cold, flu, or other illness
To enhance contemplative, artistic focus	During physical exercise
To help yourself wake up in the mornings	To fall asleep at bedtime; when having insomnia
To feel present, alive, and protected	When "out of" your body
To strengthen integrity in conflicts or others' manipulations, mirroring, or projection	When stuck in traffic or standing in a long line
To feel your authentic self	When you live in your head
For creative focus on projects	When talking obsessively or compulsively
To increase your ability to engage your consciousness	When you feel hysterical or hypersensitive
To increase a feeling of being "whole"	In situations with disarming potential
To release unwanted energy from your space	When pulled over by the police for speeding
To distinguish your energy from others'	To maintain boundaries in conflicts or others' manipulations, mirroring, or projection
When unusually overemotional	When not in the present time or place
To create a place for your spirit to feel comfortable in your body	When overanalyzing or confused
When you feel overwhelmed and incapable	For constructive, concentrated focus
When you act as a victim or perpetrator	When feeling static in your body
When other people unduly influence your thoughts or decisions	To strengthen grounding and boundaries
To clear out feelings of deadness	

LIFE FORCE	EARTH ENERGY
When you feel empty and separate from the earth and its beings	When experiencing cold feet are unable to feel your feet
When objectivity, neutrality, and compassion for self and others are compromised	When your body and spirit feel disconnected
When competing physically or mentally	When you sense only the upper part of your body
To get an unpleasant task completed	When not aware of your lower body
To cleanse out other people's energy	When you feel lopsided or asymmetrical
To be the "life of the party"	When you feel disconnected
When your hands ache or are cold	If you feel you are spinning, moving too fast, or racing like a car idling too high
When you need a boost of energy to get through the day	When pulsing with activity but unable to get focused
When you feel weakened by and disinterested in your surroundings	After working or focusing intensely for long periods without a break
When your spirit feels diminished	In anticipation of or during unpleasant activity
When your internal forces feel weak	After discordant activities
When bad habits and choices rule your decisions	During an emergency
	To soothe a tired or crying baby

LIFE-FORCE AND EARTH ENERGY: ENHANCING AND WEAKENING

Look at the lists of activities on the following pages and note which are familiar and which are unfamiliar. The activities on the "Weaken" side are the ones to avoid in your pursuit of well-being. A dedication to health demands that you pay attention to those situations and people that cause dis-ease — and then avoid them! The activities on the "Enhance" side are the ones to engage in to sustain your health and well-being.

ACTIVITIES AND THINGS THAT...	
ENHANCE LIFE-FORCE AND EARTH ENERGY	**WEAKEN LIFE-FORCE AND EARTH ENERGY**
Creative expression	Driving on freeways
Bright, sunny days	Working in an unhealthy environment
Being in nature or around flowers; gardening	Being under fluorescent lighting
Color, art, music, and reading good books	Artificial heating and cooling systems
A meeting of people for spiritual community	Hermetically sealed spaces
Completion of tasks and goals	Environments where there is stasis — where nothing ever changes
Good nutritional supplements	Alcohol, worry, stress, loud people, and crowds
Sleeping well	A long to-do list but no goal-setting list
Rest, play, and vacation time	Lack of water, vitamins, food, or sleep
Helping people; good friendships	Not enough play or vacation time
Family, love, children, and pets	Being sick or in pain
Orderly, beautiful environments	Physical exhaustion
Sharing, optimism, exploring, and learning	Stressed-out people; arguments; frustration
Slow, conscious breathing	Hearing dissonant music
Inner spiritual communication	Dealing with children when they fight
Exercise, dancing, sports, and sexual activities	Spending too much time at the computer
Being with people who have good energy	Watching television news; reading the newspaper
Relaxing at home	Interacting with unbalanced egos; inauthentic power; invalidation; control; anger
Acting and living from truth and integrity	Lack of exercise being physically stagnant
Acting from "I know" and "I trust"	
Drinking, bathing, or swimming in water	

ENHANCE LIFE-FORCE AND EARTH ENERGY	WEAKEN LIFE-FORCE AND EARTH ENERGY
Meditation with a magnet	Lack of faith; self-doubt
Opening the feet chakras	Spiritual and corporeal laziness
Sacred healing rituals	Doing only for others without self-regard
Self-love, trust, and hope	Acting from "I think" or "I should"
Positive human connection	Being in your head too much
Aromatherapy; nature smells	Too much coffee or sugar
Good connection/communication with loved ones	Lack of emotional boundaries
	Fear, anxiety, or worry
Inspirational books, music, and movies	Creating personal roadblocks
Whatever makes you feel happy and alive	Under- or overestimating the time, commitment, or energy you have to share with others and for projects
Consciousness, integrity, and joy	Repressed anger or sadness
Sharing gifts of love and caring	Blame and judgment of self or others
Eating healthy, vital food	Internalizing negative energy and thoughts
Humor and laughter	
A regular meditation practice	Being in enclosed community places: grocery stores, malls, or movie theaters
	Believing media communications without discretion
	Being indoors too long; lack of nature contact

Journaling

Think about the items on the preceding lists and how they relate to your life. I believe that the optimum practice of health for a sensitive person is to know the answer to these two questions:

1. Who tends to deplete or weaken your life-force and earth energy?

2. Who honors you and allows you to interact with them while maintaining the harmony of your life-force and earth energy?

You can explore these two questions in your journal. Your Intuition Medicine health practice is to listen to, trust, and follow through with what your intuition tells you to do when you are around depleting personalities, and to spend more time with those who honor you.

When you feel ready to begin the process of self-healing, proceed to the next chapter, "The Life-Force and Earth-Energy Meditation Practice."

I trust that this chapter has given you an awareness of your life-force and earth energy and the motivation to pursue being your own best healer. You deserve to live in a body of health every day.

Chapter 9

THE LIFE-FORCE AND EARTH-ENERGY
MEDITATION PRACTICE

The body is the temple of life.
Energy is the force of life.
Spirit is the governor of life.

— Lao-tzu

*I*n this chapter, I introduce you to life-force and earth-energy meditations that enable you to contribute more positively in relationships and
to experience a new way of belonging through increased vitality, joy, and
inner peace. When you are connected to the earth, your awareness is
heightened and you stay in the present moment. Earth energy has a healing resonance that moves through your body and stabilizes you in situations that feel threatening. Life-force energy, as it moves through your
body, supports you in feeling like yourself and helps you feel stronger
and more able to handle life's situations.

The life-force and earth-energy meditations give you a simple, powerful tool that vitalizes you with healing energy. This is the core healing
practice of the Intuition Medicine model, so this chapter includes several
instructional choices to insure that at least a few will appeal to you. You
do not need to practice with all of these sections, but do try at least the
contemplative meditation, which is the cornerstone of the intuitive healing process. In time and with practice, you will want to work with all the

sections in this chapter, as each one gives you a new perspective on bringing energy and balance to your life.

Once you master this skill of self-healing, you will have a direct and endless source of health energy. With practice, you will feel your life force and the earth's energy all day long; this is your daily dose of body-of-health living.

Contemplative Meditations

I offer two meditations here. The first meditation works solely with earth energy and is a good one to practice for relaxation during stressful times. The second meditation combines life force and earth energy, and is a complete self-healing meditation.

You may choose to do the two meditations one after the other, or just do the first one as a separate and complete meditation. Afterward, take time to reflect on your experiences with each meditation. As a guide for your learning, answer the post-meditation questions, making notes in your journal. As you take the time to develop and become fluent in the language of intuition, you are developing your wisdom voice.

Earth-Energy Meditation

- Close your eyes. Bring your attention into your head and find a quiet, still place; be there. Rest your attention in your meditation sanctuary. (See the Meditation Sanctuary illustration on page 75.)

- Come into communication with yourself in your meditation sanctuary. Greet yourself; listen to and feel your inner voice.

- Begin to focus on your breathing. Bring air in through your nose, exhale through your mouth, and continue to breathe in this way for one minute. Focus on your breathing and release all other thoughts.

- Drop your energy and emotions low to the ground. Sense the force of gravity pulling your body to the center of the earth. Hold this feeling for one minute.

- With feeling and intention, visualize the energy at your lower back and the base of your spine being pulled downward by gravity. Now feel the energy throughout your body dropping low to the ground and flowing downward, pulled by gravity.

- With your attention in your meditation sanctuary, affirm that you would like to see and know a symbol that represents your grounding. Trust the first knowing and insight that you receive. Use this grounding symbol, and visualize that symbol anchoring your body into the core of the earth. Feel yourself dropping your grounding anchor symbol deep into the earth.

- Feel the pull of this energy force. Be centered in your meditation sanctuary. Hold that feeling for a minute.

- Expand the grounding symbol and the feeling of gravity pulling your entire body into the earth, from the top of your head down to your feet. Energy follows your thought and your intention; simply affirm that your grounding field is expanding to the width of your body. Hold that feeling for a moment.

- Breathe in through your nose and exhale through your mouth. Focus your attention in your meditation sanctuary. From that point of perception, intuitively scan your body; sense and see the areas where you are holding on to tension, stress, or blocked energy. Visualize the force of gravity moving through those areas, dissolving the blocks, and gently moving them down into the earth. Take some time to move through this diagnostic and cleansing meditation.

- Come into communication with yourself and be in the center of your meditation sanctuary, affirming your intention to listen to and trust your intuition.

- Open your feet chakras, which are located at the soles of your feet. Your chakras open and close like the pupils of your eyes.

- Feel the pulse of the earth's electromagnetic current below your feet. Visualize pulling this earth energy up into your feet chakras and filling your feet. Begin to direct this energy up your legs, saturating your legs with earth energy. Direct the earth-energy flow to the bottom of your back and spine at your first chakra, then drop the energy through your grounding field and back into the earth.

- Imagine a circular flow of earth energy moving from the core of the earth, pulsing up through your feet, legs, and pelvis, and flowing back down into the earth. Meditate on this circular flow of earth energy for a minute.

- Visualize your body being bathed in this magnetic healing current. This earth-energy current will continue to flow throughout your body as you sit in quiet meditation.

- Hold this feeling for a full minute or more.

Life-Force and Earth-Energy Meditation

- Begin with the earth-energy meditation described above.

- From your meditation sanctuary, and in intuitive inquiry, affirm seeing or sensing a symbol, color, tone, or other representation of your life-force healing energy. Trust the first information that comes to you. Visualize placing your life-force symbol above you, within your aura. Visualize this symbol generating, toning, and amplifying your highest current of personal healing energy. Sense that feeling and hold it for a moment.

- Visualize directing your life-force energy into your body through your seventh chakra at the top of your head (see the Grounding, Life-Force Energy and Earth Energy illustrations on pages 114–115). Affirm that your life-force energy pulses down the back of your body and follows your spine down to its base, where your first chakra is located.

- At your first chakra, the earth-energy pulse naturally blends with your life-force healing energy and begins to resonate in a unified field of healing current. Direct this blended energy up your spine and through the front of your body.

- When the energy reaches your neck, send some of the energy across your shoulders, down your arms, and out your open hand chakras into your aura.

- Direct the rest of the current up your neck, through your head, and out the top of your head. The energy flows like a fountain of water out the top of your seventh chakra and showers throughout your aura, forming a cocoon of life-force energy around your body.

- Repeat these steps until you see and feel the current of life-force and earth energy flowing easily.

- Now affirm directing your life-force and earth energy throughout all your systems: your physical body, chakras, aura, and grounding. Do this several times until you feel full of your light, warmth, pulse, or another recognition of your life-force energy.

- Feel your life force in your hands. Open your hand chakras 100 percent and visualize currents of your life force amplifying in your hands. Hold this feeling for a moment until your hands warm up or feel tingly or you experience a pulse or another recognition that your hands hold the current of your personal signature life-force energy.

- Visualize any specific area where you would like to do healing, and lay your hands on that area. Direct a current of life force into that area with the intention of saturating it and raising its level of healing energy.

- Visualize a blueprint of all your systems. Fill the blueprint with your life-force and earth energy. Affirm that health and harmony resonate within the imagery of all your systems in the blueprint. Hold that intention for a minute.

- Reach out and pull your ideal-health blueprint into your body, ground it through your body, and anchor it into the earth.

- Bring your attention into your meditation sanctuary and greet yourself. Come into communication with yourself.

- Within your meditation sanctuary, affirm that you are receiving a gift of your personal wisdom. Hold that gift in a quiet, still place for a moment.

- Be present in your meditation sanctuary. Hold this body-of-health healing space for a minute or more.

Observational Practices

Post-Meditation Questions

To stimulate your skills in clairvoyance and knowing, reflect on these questions while centered in your meditation sanctuary:

1. What did you learn about your life force and the earth's energy?

2. Note the percentages of each of these energies that were running through your body.

3. How did you sense the life-force and earth energy?

4. Was life force or earth energy a familiar feeling?

5. Was this meditation evocative of certain moods or particular events in your life?

6. Did you see colors, patterns, or symbols?

7. Did you sense areas in your energy space being filled with vitality?

8. Which areas of your body were in need of cleansing and upgrading?

9. Which areas of your body needed more vitality?

Reflection

Look at the lists on the following pages, then count the number of "in harmony" and "out of harmony" experiences that are familiar to you. Use these lists as a diagnostic tool to tell you when you need to practice your life force and earth energy meditations — and when to congratulate yourself for being full of life and health.

LIFE-FORCE AND EARTH-ENERGY EXPERIENCE

WHEN IN HARMONY, YOU...	WHEN OUT OF HARMONY, YOU...
Feel "I know who I am"	Lose your sense of identity
Feel alive and well	Feel tired and lethargic
Experience palpable consciousness	Feel separate from life
Have a large experience of life	Feel isolated
Are calm, focused, assertive, lucid, and strong	Are frazzled, overly emotional, or unclear
Feel heightened creativity and personal power	Find it difficult to accomplish things
Are creative and inspired	Feel your creativity stifled
Have a unique feeling of lightness and joy	Feel anxiety, stress, or that you are stuck in your head
Are centered and present in your body	Feel numb or devoid of emotions or body awareness
Have plenty of energy to handle whatever comes up	Are unproductive; little things take too much time and a lot of effort
Find that your day goes smoothly and easily	Complain, whine, or feel impatient
Are productive, calm or excited, confident, and vital	Need bed and a trashy novel/video
Feel in harmony with others	Find that everything looks bland or lifeless
Receive smiles, compliments, and recognition	Have no inspiration; feel unmotivated or overwhelmed
Are in the present moment, with no angst or worry	Feel tense, nervous, scattered, scared, confused, spacey, or hurried
Feel compassion for yourself and others	Are out of touch with your physical/emotional needs
Have an authentic feeling of your personal center	Feel resistance; things just do not work
Know how to speak, act, and listen from a place of wisdom	Look for a safe place to be
Experience flow and a state of grace	Find it difficult to relax or be at ease
	Have constant mundane concerns
	Make decisions constantly
	Cannot get out of bed in the morning
	Have difficulty completing or starting tasks

WHEN IN HARMONY, YOU...	WHEN OUT OF HARMONY, YOU...
Accept your time and place in life	Are generally restless or listless
Feel clear, focused, present, energized, and stabilized	Feel that outside forces control your life
Feel a source of infinite, boundless physical energy	Are rattled by life
Know without thinking	Are easily agitated and depressed
Feel nourished from within	Lack trust
Are happy without a need to be perfect	Say stupid things or act ungraciously
Trust yourself	Do things that do not express your authentic self
Feel vital, with a calm, present attention	Feel dispassionate about life
Feel in control of life	
Experience synchronicity in life	
Feel life-supporting	
Feel at home wherever you are	
Feel a deep sense of calm	

Daily-Living Tips

- Begin to notice the flow of earth energy and life force in your body. Intuit the times during your day when you need more earth energy or more life force.

- During your day, adjust the flow of earth energy and life force in your body as needed to bring yourself into a state of well-being and vitality.

Experiments: Try This!

- When you receive acupuncture, chiropractic, massage, or other healing work, visualize earth and life-force energies pulsing through your body during the treatment. Do the same when swimming, running, or doing any type of exercise. The benefit to your physical strength and well-being is enormous — and it multiplies the feel-good experience!

- When you are agitated or nervous, find a piece of earth to lie down on. Close your eyes and visualize earth energy rising up and saturating your body. Continue doing this until you feel peaceful.

Affirmations: Repeat Often

- I am abundant in my love of self and others.
- I practice compassion with myself and others.
- My creativity is expansive.
- I see goodness in myself and in the world around me.
- I practice truth.
- I trust my intuition.
- I operate in life with ease and grace.

Trust

You already have life-force and earth energy within you, and you already know this information. Trust the intelligence of your body, as it has been evolving into a higher state of wellness for eons. Trust that your spirit is wise and knows how to live with love and health. Cherish being alive.

Chapter 10

THE CHAKRA SYSTEM:
PHYSICAL AND SPIRITUAL HEALTH

The new medical science will be outstandingly built upon the science of the chakra centers, and upon this knowledge all diagnosis and possible cure will be based.

— Alice A. Bailey

$\mathcal{S}$piritual wisdom, physical health, and well-being are coded within the chakras. The unbroken, continuous symbolic voice of the chakra has been kept alive as it passed from our ancestors through all generations of humankind. The secret knowledge of the chakras is taught in the tenets of the religious and esoteric orders of the Jesuits, Freemasons, Rosicrucians, and Theosophists. The earliest evidence of chakra symbolism from European cave paintings and artifacts is about thirty-five thousand years old.[1]

The etymology of human language is found in symbols. The ability to attach meaning to objects and observations requires abstract intuitive thought and is at the root of human culture. From the ancient universal symbol of the chakra to the recent alphabetic symbols, transmission of information has been an intrinsic part of our survival and evolution.

Many people consider the "whirling wheel" symbol to be the earliest human ideogram. *Chakra* is a Sanskrit word that means "wheel," and the human chakras are typically described as being configured like wheels. Chakra symbolism was painted in Paleolithic caves and is found worldwide in all cultures and countries.

141

A World of Chakras

Many people consider the "whirling wheel" symbol to be the earliest human ideogram. *Chakra* is a Sanskrit word that means "wheel," and the human chakras are typically described as being configured like wheels. Chakra symbolism was painted on Paleolithic caves, and is found worldwide in all cultures and countries.

Our world is filled with chakra symbols, depicted in numerous artistic renditions. The chakra ideogram is displayed as: the main symbol of the East Indian religion, Jainism; the logo of the Indira Gandhi National Centre for the Arts; a central Balinese religious symbol; the logo for the Singapore Red Swastika Hospital (the Red Cross organization of Asia); the seal of the Theosophical society; and the central symbol on flags of British crown possessions and the old national flag of Sicily (as a triskelion — one of the oldest continually used government symbols). Decorative chakra depictions are found universally in art and architecture: at the temple of the Oracle of Delphi; within Mayan temple walls; in Christian symbology, in the crowns of the four-and-twenty elders seated at the throne of God; in Celtic glyphs; in Aboriginal walkabout paintings; on Egyptian tarot cards; on the floor of a fourth-century Algerian basilica; on ancient Israeli synagogue floors; on the cathedral floor at Chartres, France; as the Chakra Labyrinth in Oshkosh, Wisconsin; in the garden at Grace Cathedral in San Francisco; on the crown of the statute of the Snake Goddess at Knossos; on the entrance gates to Calcutta; and painted on the wall of Jesus' tomb in Holy Sepulture Cathedral in Jerusalem.

Variations of the symbol are found in ceremonial artifacts: Native American sand paintings and burial mounds, pottery of the Ahwahnee, medicine healing dolls of the Navajo, banners of the Zuni, Hopi Kivas, Mayan and Aztec masks, the mandalas of Tibetan monks, and Christian vestments found in Roman catacombs.

In India, it is a sign of good health to shave a child's head and draw a chakra symbol on the top of the head.[2] Legend says that a chakra symbol was found as a birthmark on the feet of all Buddhas. The Buddha is described as having many designs on the palms of his hands, one of which is a svastika.[3] The word "swastika" is taken from the Sanskrit *svastika*, meaning "to be well."

CHAKRA LOCATIONS

In the Intuition Medicine model, our practice focuses on seven major chakras and three sets of minor chakras (see both the Chakra System Definitions illustration on page 145 and the Endocrine System and Chakra Correspondences illustration on page 146). The seven main chakras and corresponding endocrine glands are:

1. the first chakra, located at the base of the spine about two inches below the navel (relays energy-information to the adrenal glands);

2. the second chakra, located at the navel (relays energy-information to the gonads);

3. the third chakra, located at the abdomen (relays energy-information to the pancreas);

4. the fourth chakra, located in the center of the chest at the sternum (relays energy-information to the thymus gland);

5. the fifth chakra, located at the cleft of the throat (relays energy-information to the thyroid gland);

6. the sixth chakra, located in the center of the forehead (relays energy-information to the pineal gland);

7. and the seventh chakra, located on the top of the head — the "soft spot" on newborns (relays energy-information to the pituitary gland).

The minor chakras in our energy model are:

• the feet chakras, located on the soles of the feet;

• the hand chakras, located in the center of the palms;

• and the telepathic chakras, located around the eyes, at each temple, behind each ear.

Think of the chakras and endocrine glands working together to transform spiritual energy into physical energy. The endocrine glands function as the first physical receptor sites for the spiritual energy of the chakras. The endocrine glands act as transducers that tap into human beings' potential to evolve through the combined action of physical healing and the wisdom forces of the universe. When you manage chakra-endocrine system energy, a coherent pathway for your spiritual journey manifests.

CHAKRA DEFINITIONS: SACRED CIRCLES

Chakras are like computer chips, programmed for specific data reception, storage, and transmission. Your chakras are programmed with information input from many sources: hereditary, cellular, karmic, cosmological, and universal consciousness. This data is continually being updated, sorted, referenced, added to, and deleted, consciously and unconsciously. Your self-healing practice allows you to be the conscious data processor of your chakra information.

Rather than assessing health situations as either "healthy" or "diseased," I suggest that healers think about the inherent spiritual or emotional learning within the situation and refer to the dis-ease as its by-product. When you feel or experience something that might be labeled as "dark" or "diseased," consider recognizing that information or situation as a waiting lesson of wisdom. Practice intuitive inquiry from your meditation sanctuary, asking, "What can I learn from this dis-ease?" or "What is the lesson in this unhappy episode in my life?" These inner-voice questions evoke information that holds the answers for healing. The more you apply this approach, the faster the information, learning, results, and healing will occur.

The first chakra, or root chakra, located at the base of the spine, synthesizes information on physical health, basic survival needs, financial issues, and career concerns, as well as issues concerning children, siblings, parents, family, and extended family. With a first chakra in healthy operation, you feel grounded, in your body, and connected to the earth. You can provide for your basic survival needs, and you maintain a healthy outlook on your career pursuits and your family life. A first chakra in

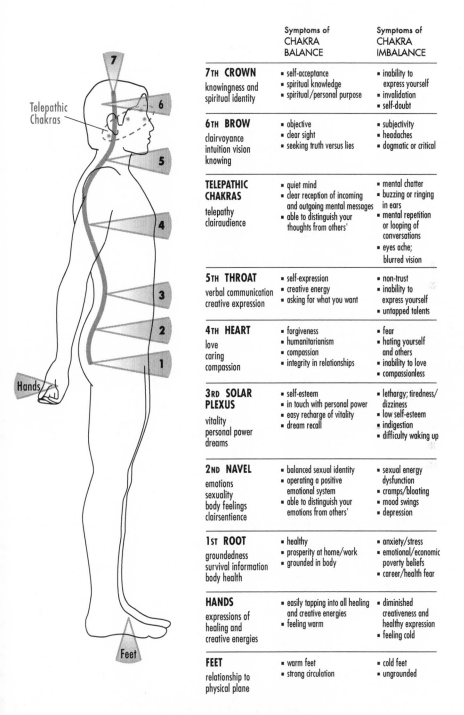

	Symptoms of CHAKRA BALANCE	Symptoms of CHAKRA IMBALANCE
7TH CROWN knowingness and spiritual identity	• self-acceptance • spiritual knowledge • spiritual/personal purpose	• inability to express yourself • invalidation • self-doubt
6TH BROW clairvoyance intuition vision knowing	• objective • clear sight • seeking truth versus lies	• subjectivity • headaches • dogmatic or critical
TELEPATHIC CHAKRAS telepathy clairaudience	• quiet mind • clear reception of incoming and outgoing mental messages • able to distinguish your thoughts from others'	• mental chatter • buzzing or ringing in ears • mental repetition or looping of conversations • eyes ache; blurred vision
5TH THROAT verbal communication creative expression	• self-expression • creative energy • asking for what you want	• non-trust • inability to express yourself • untapped talents
4TH HEART love caring compassion	• forgiveness • humanitarianism • compassion • integrity in relationships	• fear • hating yourself and others • inability to love • compassionless
3RD SOLAR PLEXUS vitality personal power dreams	• self-esteem • in touch with personal power • easy recharge of vitality • dream recall	• lethargy; tiredness/dizziness • low self-esteem • indigestion • difficulty waking up
2ND NAVEL emotions sexuality body feelings clairsentience	• balanced sexual identity • operating a positive emotional system • able to distinguish your emotions from others'	• sexual energy dysfunction • cramps/bloating • mood swings • depression
1ST ROOT groundedness survival information body health	• healthy • prosperity at home/work • grounded in body	• anxiety/stress • emotional/economic poverty beliefs • career/health fear
HANDS expressions of healing and creative energies	• easily tapping into all healing and creative energies • feeling warm	• diminished creativeness and healthy expression • feeling cold
FEET relationship to physical plane	• warm feet • strong circulation	• cold feet • ungrounded

CHAKRA SYSTEM DEFINITIONS

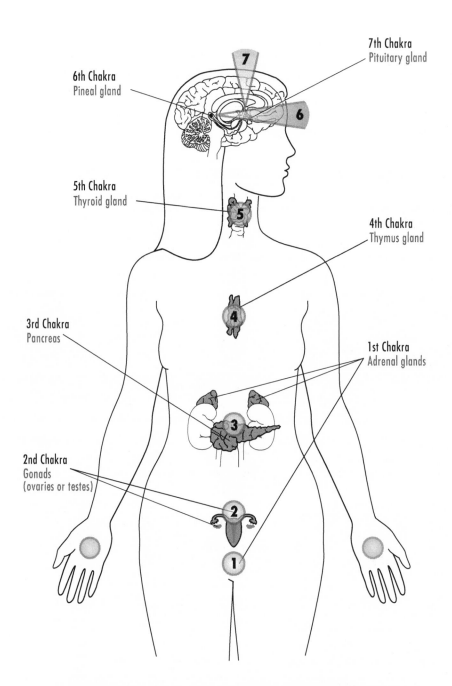

7th Chakra
Pituitary gland

6th Chakra
Pineal gland

5th Chakra
Thyroid gland

4th Chakra
Thymus gland

3rd Chakra
Pancreas

1st Chakra
Adrenal glands

2nd Chakra
Gonads
(ovaries or testes)

ENDOCRINE SYSTEM AND CHAKRA CORRESPONDENCES

lesson-learning mode can cause nervous, anxious, fearful feelings, a lowered sense of well-being, job worries, and family and financial stress. Areas of the physical body affected by the first chakra can include the lower back, hips, legs, intestines, and adrenal glands.

The second chakra, located at the navel, is the energetic center for emotion and sexuality. With a second chakra in healthy operation, you experience a range of appropriate emotions from joy to sadness, express your own emotions in a harmonious manner, and engage in healthy sexual relationships. A second chakra in lesson-learning mode can cause dramatic mood swings, depression, overwhelming feelings of empathy, and sexual dysfunction. Areas of the physical body affected by the second chakra can include the reproductive system, intestinal and digestive systems, sciatic nerve, and lower back.

The third chakra, located at the solar plexus, is your personal power center. With a third chakra in healthy operation, you feel full of vitality and strength, you wake up feeling refreshed and ready to start your day, you gracefully engage in power struggles at work and at home, and you remember your dreams upon waking. A third chakra in lesson-learning mode can cause lethargy, morning fatigue, debilitating power struggles, and associated anger, low self-esteem, and nightmares. Areas of the physical body affected by the third chakra include the stomach, spleen, pancreas, gallbladder, adrenals, and middle of the back.

The fourth chakra, located in the middle of the chest, is the center of compassion and love for self and others. A fourth chakra in healthy operation allows you to validate yourself with a sense of self-love and care, maintain a healthy balance between your own emotional needs and those of others, and feel and express love, altruism, care, and compassion for others. The ancient wisdom practices define love as emotion without duality. A fourth chakra in lesson-learning mode can cause feelings of loss, grief, anger, and hatred, and the inability to feel or express love for yourself or others. Areas of the physical body affected by the fourth chakra are the heart, lungs, thymus, respiratory system, and middle of the back.

The fifth chakra, located at the throat, is the center for communication and creative expression. A fifth chakra in healthy operation allows for positive, productive communication with others. You are able to communicate clearly and comfortably, and you can express your personal creativity in the world. A fifth chakra in lesson-learning mode can cause fear of expression, inability to speak your personal truth, and unwillingness to recognize and utilize your creative abilities. Areas of the physical body affected by the fifth chakra are the throat, neck, shoulders, arms, mouth, nose, and thyroid gland.

The sixth chakra, located in the center of the forehead, is the center for intuitive perception, clairvoyance, and intuition. A sixth chakra in healthy operation allows you to recognize and utilize your intuitive abilities, clearly perceive people and situations, and maintain a positive, effective balance between intuitive and analytical thought. A sixth chakra in lesson-learning mode can lead to a dogmatic, judgmental, or subjective point of view, overreliance on logic and analytical thought, and an inability to see the truth in people and situations. Areas of the physical body affected by this chakra can include the face and head, eyes, ears, nose, and the back of the head.

The seventh or crown chakra, located on the top of the head, is the center of your personal spiritual identity. A seventh chakra in healthy operation allows for a well-developed sense of self, a strong connection to your personal spirituality, and a clear sense of your life path. A seventh chakra in lesson-learning mode can lead to a diminished sense of self, an inability to take control of your life, and unwillingness to recognize and connect with the spiritual element in your life. Physical areas affected by the seventh chakra can include the top and back of the head, the brain, and the pituitary gland.

The hand chakras, located in the middle of your palms, are centers for expressing your creativity in the world and for developing a sense of psychometry. Hand chakras in healthy operation allow you to freely manifest your creative ideas in the world and utilize your energy-healing ability. Hand chakras in lesson-learning mode can cause blocked creative expression and limit your energy-healing skill. Physical areas affected by these minor chakras can include fingers, hands, wrists, forearms, and shoulder joints.

The feet chakras, located on the bottoms of your feet, are your connecting points to the physical world. Feet chakras in healthy operation allow you to sense your relationship with the earth, ground fully into your body, and walk with physical balance and grace. Feet chakras in lesson-learning mode can cause clumsiness, impaired balance, and disconnection from the earth and your body. Physical areas affected by these minor chakras can include the sciatic nerve, feet, and legs.

The telepathic chakras are located around your eyes, at your temples, and behind your ears. These are the centers for mental communication. Telepathic chakras in healthy operation allow you to send and receive nonverbal messages as needed. Telepathic chakras in lesson-learning mode can be the cause of overwhelming chatter in your head, an inability to mentally or visually focus, and difficulty getting to sleep. Physical areas affected by these minor chakras include the head, eyes, ears, nose, and mouth.

Recognize and interpret the energetic, physical, and emotional elements of each chakra and allow yourself to sense when your chakras are in healthy mode and when they are in lesson-learning mode. As your intuitive perception increases, you will experience the value of meditation to maintain the homeostasis of your chakras (see details in chapter 11). You will also identify the lesson-learning symptoms earlier and ask questions that give you wisdom keys.

CHAKRAS ARE THREE-DIMENSIONAL

If the doors of perception were cleansed, everything would appear to man as it is — infinite.[4]

— William Blake

You can use gadgets from your kitchen and a toy box to give you an image of how a chakra looks and functions. Gather a funnel, a toy pinwheel, and a stainless-steel vegetable steamer (the type that allows its "petals" to pop open like a flower and expands or folds to adjust to various pot sizes). Hold the funnel in your hands; feel the shape and look at the configuration. The shape is three-dimensional, like a chakra; there is a smaller opening at the bottom and a larger opening at the top, corresponding to the healthy apertures at the back (bottom) and front (top) of a chakra. Now pick up the vegetable steamer and observe its shape and movement potential. Place the vegetable steamer over one of your chakras, with the bottom of the steamer flat against your body and the area that opens wide facing away from your body. Opening and closing the vegetable steamer mimics the aperture motion of the chakras. When both the vegetable steamer and your chakras are in good working order you should be able to easily adjust the openness. Another movement within the chakras is like that of a pinwheel. Blow on the pinwheel; if it is in good working order, it spins easily without any glitches. This is the movement within the center of your chakras — the propulsion action that receives and relays the energy-information as it enters and exits the chakra. Finally, take all three gadgets and put them together to build a chakra. Place the vegetable steamer inside the funnel, and the pinwheel inside the vegetable steamer, and blow on the pinwheel. These three gadgets create a multidimensional moving depiction of a chakra!

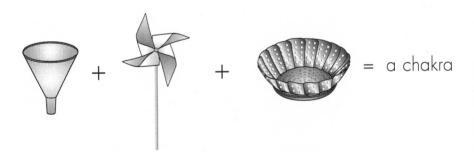

SYMBOLIC METAPHOR FOR THE WORKINGS OF A CHAKRA

Using this model to further clarify the visualization of a chakra, the narrow point at the bottom of the funnel connects to the energy channels that carry life force and other energies; the wide top part of the funnel is the saucerlike energy depression on the surface of your skin — the location point where an acupuncture needle would be inserted.

Your chakras are not the size of the funnel, vegetable steamer, or pinwheel. A chakra is approximately 1 inch across, or the size of a U.S. quarter. Chakras at times feel larger or smaller; in those instances, you are sensing the radial flow of the energy field rather than the skin-surface contact point of the chakra. When you sense that a chakra is emitting energy farther out, this is what I call a "dialed-up" or larger opening of that chakra. Conversely, I refer to a close-to-the-body flow of the chakra energy-field as a "dialed-down" or smaller opening of the chakra. As with the dilation of the iris of your eye, the aperture dials up or down, which influences its perspective, reception, and function. A wide range of activities in which you might choose to focus on opening or closing your chakras is described in the "When to 'Dial Down' or 'Open Up' Your Chakras" chart in appendix 2.

The opening and closing "movement" is a result of the intensity, flux, and propulsion of the chakra energy field. The spin is influenced by energy as it revolves through the chakra, in the same way that the rotor of an electric motor turns when positive and negative currents (life-force and earth energy) are directed into it. There is a caveat about using a pinwheel to visualize the spin of a chakra. A toy pinwheel typically moves counterclockwise, while most people's chakras north of the equator move clockwise, and those south of the equator move counterclockwise. If you are north of the equator, look down at your body and imagine that your chakras are clocks; the chakra spin moves in the direction that the clock hands rotate. You can observe a similar action when flushing a toilet: north of the equator, the water moves clockwise, while south of the equator, water moves in a counterclockwise spiral.

Frequency measurements done on the bioelectrical activity of the chakra "spin" discovered that its average range is between 100 and 1,600 cycles per second. To put this into perspective, electrical activity associated with biological function ranges from 0 to 250 cycles per second. Interestingly, each time I give a lecture on the chakra system — and before I state my theory on chakra spin — I ask the students in which direction they experience their chakras spinning. Without exception, all those students who were born north of the equator say that their chakras spin clockwise, and those born south of the equator say that their chakras spin counterclockwise.

SPIRITUAL JOURNEY OF THE SEVEN

Resonating to the vibration of "seven," the Classical Labyrinth has a direct correlation with the primary chakras, tones on the scale, and colors of the rainbow.[5]

— Reverend Lauren Artess

Metaphysical scholars have noted the correlation in numerous art, artifacts, and architecture between the number seven and the seven major chakras. For example, labyrinths are symbolic representations of a spiritual wisdom journey and are found throughout the world at sacred sites. I theorize that the ancient labyrinths are coded maps used to understand the flux and flow of energy-information in the chakra system, similar to our modern physics equations or electrical engineering diagrams. My intuitive understanding of the chakra system is analogous to numerous scientific formulations and ancient healing practices. Physics, for example, says that ions flow to the body like lightning to a lightning rod, by attraction to the points of least resistance. Chakra areas have decreased resistance, so electrical currents flow predominantly through these points into the body.

According to Chinese medicine, ayurvedic medicine, neuroscience, biomolecular science, and energy medicine, energy is transmitted into the chakras via a relay system. The energy-information is received by a programmed receptor chakra site. For example, love information enters the fourth chakra, sexual information the second chakra, and so forth. This energy-information is relayed to the corresponding endocrine gland, which is activated by the energy impulse to secrete a mood- and health-altering hormone. The hormonal secretion signal is registered by the neuropeptides, then carried through the bodywide system. Neuropeptides are the molecules most closely aligned with emotions. This energy-field relay communication is an intelligent, autonomic network system.[6] Our body, mind, and spirit are directly affected by the health of our chakra system. When you manage chakra-endocrine energy, a coherent pathway manifests, unfolding your spiritual labyrinth within your body.

A sixty-year-old dentist and first-year Intuition Medicine practitioner came to a deep appreciation of the chakra system:

Each chakra is its own world. Through my meditation practice, I have a greater understanding of how information and emotions are processed and stored. I see this internal landscape as a key to my spiritual and personal growth. I feel that the work with my chakra system is going to be a lifelong process of learning and healing. I am very grateful for this information.

The Mystical Number Seven

Many traditions refer to the seven chakras using various symbols. Author Manly P. Hall refers to the mystical representation of seven chakras in the Bible:

When related to the Eastern system of metaphysics, these seven churches represent the chakras, or nerve ganglia along the spine. In the fourth and fifth chapters [of the Bible], St. John describes the throne of God upon which sat the Holy One. About the throne were twenty-four lesser seats, upon which sat twenty-four elders arrayed in white garments and wearing crowns of gold. "And out of the throne proceeded lightenings and thunderings and voices: there were seven lamps of fire burning before the throne which are the seven spirits of God." He who sat upon the throne held in his right hand a book sealed with seven seals, which no man in heaven or earth had been found worthy to open. Then appeared a Lamb ... having seven rays and seven eyes.[7]

CHAKRAS AND HEALTH

Physical and psychological health are correlated with the chakras. You can trace physical feelings from chakra points to physical sites that receive, translate, and relay energy through the body. Worry is a major cause of energy-related health issues. If you worry about a job interview, for example, you may get a stomachache and a headache. The energy enters the third chakra (which represents personal power) and the sixth chakra (perception), then travels to the corresponding endocrine glands (pancreas and pineal), which in turn alter your mood via hormonal secretions and thus affect the health of your entire body (see the Endocrine System and Chakra Correspondences illustration on page 146).

A chakra is a focal point for the reception and transmission of energy. Energy is information. Energy-information takes form in conscious and unconscious emotions, mental thoughts, actions, and auditory frequencies (human, mechanical, or cosmological). The reception of information via the chakras impacts your feelings, emotions, thoughts, moods, and character — often whether or not you are aware of the subtle impact of energy-information. Your practice of Intuition Medicine makes you more aware rather than less aware; you become the cause of your experience rather than being merely affected by the world around you.

Chinese medicine, unadulterated by the influence of Cartesian thought, describes the health system of acupuncture as vital energy circulating through the body on specific pathways, emerging at seven hundred points (chakras) on the skin. The pathways were mapped out thousands of years ago, before there were laboratory instruments, through direct physician observation and patient self-assessment. In Chinese medicine, a state of health indicates a free flow of vital energy throughout all the pathways and points. Originally, this healing system was a personal practice of visualization meditation, focused on healing the vital energy flow at the blocked points. As the system degraded, the next application was to engage a teacher/physician who would apply pressure to the blocked points to unblock the dis-eased energy flow.

Then followed a further degradation in which a physician would diagnose and then treat a person via acupuncture needle insertion. Electroacupuncture is a further move away from the original healing meditation practice. Acupuncture healing theory states that the chakra points on the skin are in communication with organs deep inside the body, as well as with a person's whole mental and psychological state. Changing the energy flow at these points changes the vital energy deep inside the body, bringing homeostasis to the organism.[8]

The human body is an electrophysiological instrument — a subtle sensor of energy-information. Standing outdoors, you are subject to both natural and human-made electromagnetic fields; indoors, to the currents of the electrical components within the surrounding structure. There is an interrelationship between the electrical properties in the environment and those of a living system. Since one field cannot exist within another field without interacting and the properties of the ionosphere are continuously modified by the electrical characteristics of the environment, sensitive people are no doubt affected by many "unseen" forces.[9] The energetic fluctuations of your chakras, as noted earlier, lie in a band of frequencies between 100 and 1,600 cycles per second — figures far higher than what has been found radiating from the human body. To put this into perspective, the normal frequency range of brain waves is between 0 and 100 cycles per second, with most information processes occurring between 0 and 30 cycles per second.[10]

A voltmeter is an instrument that can be used to diagnose localized physical conditions. A voltmeter can measure life force by registering it at a distance from the affected area or organ. This shows that a true energy field is being measured, not a skin-surface potential. This diagnostic method can also electrically measure the intensity of worry, grief, anger, or love in the chakras.[11] In other words, emotions can be equated with quantifiable, measurable energy.

You can also measure the life-force energy in your chakras psychometrically. Place your hands a few inches in front of a chakra (not in contact with the skin); when a chakra is blocked, stagnant, or closed, you will feel nothing psychometrically in or between your hands. If the blockage is superficial, an earth-energy flush of the chakra will usually work. If more clearing is necessary, visualize gold life-force energy to clean and clear the chakra (see the 'Health Issues Reference Chart' in appendix 1). Once you can feel energy moving freely between both hands, fill the chakra with life-force energy, intend that the back of the chakra fits snugly into the chakra, and set the chakra aperture to an appropriate openness. In your self-healing practice, you literally hold the instrument for measuring the state of your health and emotions in your body and hands.

SACRED SCIENCE OF THE CHAKRAS

Chakras continually play the movie of your life, but sometimes you need subtitles to read the story line. Your intuition is the key language for reading the chakra information script. Your living diary, the chakra system journals memories, emotions, wisdom, and healing energy.

How do you read chakra information? Intuitive insight precedes wisdom, and intuition is an essential part of the formulation of knowledge; many revolutionary discoveries arrived via "aha" knowing, the flash of insight turning on like a lightbulb over the head. Your personal insight offers experiential information that is essential to the spiritual and scientific study of subtle energy systems. Given the intangibles of conventional science and the fact that the human chakra system was not discovered in a laboratory, personal study of your chakras provides the most pragmatic information. You are the human instrument for understanding your chakras. Your sensory interaction with your human instrument is as relevant as a scientist's sensory contact with a laboratory instrument. The laws of physics cannot determine the truth about life, reality, or spirit through cognitive or materialistic scrutiny. All laws are relative, not universal. Pythagoras taught that, although the material world was subject to laws, "there is another higher state of being in which the soul would rise above the laws of the lower world."[12]

Before the seventeenth-century Western materialistic view of the world created a dichotomy between the body and the spirit, science and spirituality worked together as a unified field of study. The original theory of the unity of body and spirit has been kept alive in indigenous cultures, Eastern medicine, and spiritual traditions. Recently, a growing number of spiritually invested scientists have designed laboratory instruments that register subtle human energy and have created quantifiable experiments to test the subtle energy systems of the chakras and the aura. These Western-based, scientifically modeled studies substantiate and correlate the data from human instruments.[13] This rediscovery of the constancy of spirit is much like reinventing ancient medicine. As Harry Truman said, "The only thing new in the world is the history you don't know."[14]

A Chakra by Any Other Name

Called by many names in different cultures, traditions, and lore, "chakra" is the most generally accepted name for the energy centers of the human body. Other names include wheels of light, circles of light, vortices, Sephiroths, Fylfot, Sonnenrad, triskelions, pentacles, trees of life, solar crosses, life centers, energy points, etheric organs, nerve plexuses, thousand-petalled lotuses, Rosicrucian roses, crosses of Thor, seven lamps, seven churches, seven-circuit labyrinth, mystic maze, cosmic eggs, sacred discs, portals, dimensional doorways, sacred gateways, and svasticas.

Although the name varies among cultures and traditions, the various chakra images have been mystical symbols since antiquity (except for the more recent Nazi adaptation of the swastika). Chakra is the term we use in our practice of Intuition Medicine.

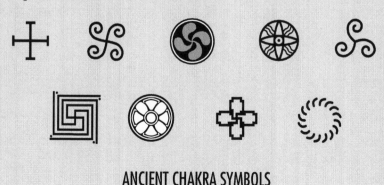

ANCIENT CHAKRA SYMBOLS

VISUALIZATION AND IMAGINATION IN MEDITATION

Using imagination to visualize the health of your chakras is good, as imagination empowers you and heightens all aspects of your intuitive sense. Healing your chakras through visualization meditation creates a vocabulary and a compilation of symbols, producing a heightened intuitive perception. With practice, you will develop a translation formula to diagnose the energy-information in your chakras.

Researchers John DeLuca and Ray Daly conducted an informative study of the brain-wave patterns of experienced meditators. They worked with practitioners of three disciplines: mindfulness meditation (no thoughts); analytical meditation (use of logical thought); and visualization meditation (use of imagination). The resulting data showed that in the visualization process, the inner contemplative concentration led to a state of transcending time, which brought a meditator to a present-time perception. In "no-thought" meditation, the practitioner was found to be acting as a channel or conduit for Divine universal energy from an external source. By contrast, in visualization meditation, the practitioner embodied that Divine energy from within. Thus, the no-thought practitioner retrieved and distributed Divine energy, while the visualization practitioner became the Divine energy.[15]

A thirty-two-year-old somatic bodyworker and first-year Intuition Medicine practitioner made the following observation:

I can't see chakras using my usual analytical mind, or — as I call it — when I am hanging out in the front of my brain. When I do give up that need to be in control and move to my meditation sanctuary, I am amazed at what I see. I recall my first glimpse of a chakra: I saw a whirling vortex of light that looked very much like a spiral galaxy. It was an amazing sight, like seeing outer space within. It gave new meaning to the phrase "As above, so below." Upon seeing this, I began to understand that energy healing is truly about energy — not the physical body per se — and, as a result, I have come to realize that energy healings need not have a "thinking" component; perhaps it is best that they do not.

WISDOM WHEELS

We don't receive wisdom; we must discover it for ourselves after a journey that no one can take us on or spare us.[16]

— Marcel Proust

I have studied the chakra system from the perspectives of the Vedic and Rosicrucian traditions and within the practice of holistic medicine. My inner guidance directed me to trust my intuition as I studied, and I would agree, disagree, or find commonality with the interpretations I was studying. Many ancient esoteric texts and recent self-help books report definitions and functions of the chakras; some are identical, some are dissimilar, and some overlap. The main aspect of those teachings that I challenge is the theory that states the "ideal color" of each chakra. I have never found or observed that any specific, standard seven colors for the seven chakras are indicative of ideal health for every person. Another aspect of chakra teachings that I challenge is the assertion that the degree of chakra openness indicates the degree of spiritual development, suggesting that the highest degree of spiritual enlightenment is seven chakras spinning at 100 percent openness. According to my own observations, such an overwhelming level of energy-information processing would drive a sensitive person into a state of insanity, aberrant possession, or a compulsive, emotional-sponge state of living.

My theory is that the concept of the standardized colors of the seven chakras and the prescription for keeping the seven chakras open at 100 percent were once valid teachings. As evolved perception contributed accumulated wisdom to the collective database of the human species, our spirit-body/intuitive-emotional systems evolved to produce a construct of individuated wisdom within the collective whole. It is to your individual wisdom that I speak. Thus, I base my Intuition Medicine work on clinical and classroom observation of clients and students and empirical study of the collected qualitative data. Thousands of human chakra systems evaluated over three decades, all with their varied permeations, contributed to the living book from which my functional definitions are derived.

The *Body of Health* definitions, data, and accumulated knowledge all summarize experiences gathered from thousands of clients and students. But, ultimately, you are your best guide in extrapolating truth from any collection of group wisdom. Direct experience aligns and grounds your wisdom. You are the spirit who lives in your body; trust what feels right to you and gives healthy results in your personal practice.

PRACTICAL CHAKRA HEALTH IN DAILY LIFE

Your chakras speak for you continuously, whether or not you are aware of this subtle talk. You can manage and greatly enhance your daily life through awareness of your chakra activity. Think of the center line of your body, with the seven major chakras lined up from the base of your spine to the top of your head, as a vertical grounding anchor. Visualize the continuous flux and flow of your life-force and earth-energy current through this grounded line of chakras. The chakra current is the carrier of the subtle-talk information.

Imagine verbally talking to a person while feeling love for her or him; your fourth chakra sends this subtle-talk information to the fourth chakra of your friend, creating a pleasant energy communication. Now imagine that you are engaged in an argument in which you feel anger being directed at you; your third chakra will receive this energy-information, and you may experience pain, pressure, or a feeling of being punched in the stomach. If you are practicing energy awareness, you can choose to close the aperture of your third chakra and thereby shut off or greatly diminish the reception of this subtle-talk dis-ease energy into your body.

As you practice active diagnostic assessment of your chakras, you will discover which are more often open and which are more often closed, which are active or quiet, and which are the dominant senders and receivers. Observe how your chakras react in various subtle-talk situations, with certain people, in different physical locations, and within groups. This is a daily energy inventory that will develop your language of intuition. Identifying this chakra information will help you manage the optimal aperture for each chakra in any situation by dialing the chakra up or down to the setting that allows you to operate in the world as a sensitive person and to maintain your health. This is a daily practice of spiritual sanity. You are a modern mystic. You are in the world, but not entirely caught up in the web of the world.

CONTEMPLATIVE CHAKRA MEDITATION

Human beings, by changing the inner attitudes of their minds, can change the outer aspects of their lives.[17]

— William James

Affirm a personal intention for your contemplative chakra practice (see chapter 11) at the start of each meditation, including specific and general goals. The three-step self-healing chakra formula is "I identify, interpret, and heal the energy of my chakras." Overall diagnostic goals for chakra meditation include identifying the energy within each chakra and the chakra system as a whole; intuiting the colors, patterns, sounds, and emotions of each chakra; and recognizing sent and received subtle-energy messages. Interpretative goals include creating a consistent energy language; this is done by writing all your perceptions, no matter how insignificant or fleeting, in your journal to evolve your personal intuition language dictionary. Utilize your intuition-language and cross-reference it with the information in this book, which includes intuitive language compiled from thousands of people. Apply this combined intuition-language dictionary to your interpretation of your chakra perceptions. Healing goals for chakra meditation include assessment of the health aperture of each chakra for situational usage, deducing the color(s) of healing for each chakra, and completely saturating the chakras with the selected healing color(s) of life-force and earth-energy.

The simplest meditations can have profound and effective healing results. In 1979, I had a clinical client who was a thirty-six-year-old woman working as a hospital X-ray technician. She was referred to me because she was experiencing persistent abdominal pain. During the previous eight months, she had been examined by four medical doctors three times a month and received multiple blood tests, X-rays, an electromyogram, a sonogram, and a spinal block. She was treated with pain pills that gradually increased in strength, all with no definitive diagnosis. In our first session, we worked intuitively with her third-chakra issues and her perceived power struggle between herself and her boss, which were blocking the spin of her third chakra. Once we had identified the energy, it easily released.

I gave her a contemplative healing prescription, which was to center her attention in her meditation sanctuary for thirty minutes each day, visualizing gold life-force and earth energy in her chakras, with emphasis on her third chakra. When she returned the next week, she reported that her pain had left the day after our session and had not returned. She felt well enough to return to work after being on leave for eight months. I advised her to continue her daily meditation. The third and last time I saw her, she was feeling well and free of pain. Ten years later, she contacted me to say hello. When I asked about her past abdominal pain, she told me that it had never recurred; whenever she began to feel her third-chakra-blockage symptoms she immediately renewed her daily thirty-minute meditations.

If healing energy is successfully focused by whatever means, it results in transformation. All true physicians seek the same thing; the chasm between alternative therapy and Western medicine is illusory. Western medicine springs from the same roots and, in the final analysis, acts through the same forces as alternative, complementary, holistic, integrative, and energy medicine. All worthwhile medical research, and every practitioner's intuition, is part of the same quest for knowledge of the same healing energy.

CHAKRAS ARE HEALTH TOOLS

*As I see it, every day you do one of two things: build health or produce
disease in yourself.*[18]

— Adelle Davis

Physical, psychological, and spiritual health depend on your practice of
self-awareness in relation to the intuitive language of your chakras.
Subtle talk, hunches, and hits — what you feel, sense, perceive, and
know — are the intuitive health tools in your Intuition Medicine bag.

Here is an observation from a forty-year-old woman who is a third-
year Intuition Medicine practitioner and a landscape architect:

*My chakra system tells the story of how I am. I can sense the opening and
closing of these amazing energy centers. Their function and health are
vital to my well-being. These energy areas of my body are a source of deep
knowledge. As I travel through my chakra journey, more of the onion is
being peeled and information is being revealed to me. For example, I
know that I let people come into my second chakra easily, which allows
them to influence my emotions and sexuality. My father connects into my
fifth chakra, so he influences my voice and creativity. But I now have the
tools to help myself — to clear out people, things, and energy in my
chakras that do not serve my highest good. And I have tools to heal myself
with my own energy.*

Reflections and Journaling

The core practice for maintaining your physical health is to pay attention to the language of your chakras. Stop for a moment and reflect
on the "In Harmony" and "Out of Harmony" lists on the following
page; as you read the lists, scan your body and notice your feelings. Your
body is always talking to you as sensation; when you pay attention, you
can interpret this sense-language.

HOW IT FEELS WHEN CHAKRAS ARE...	
IN HARMONY	**OUT OF HARMONY**
Vibrant, clear, pulsing, and active	Anxious, queasy, or painful
Rich in color, bright, and full of light	Butterflies in one's stomach
Relaxed and energized, with a sense of peace	Heartache or emotional pain
Safely containing all emotions, including the painful or sorrowful ones	Blocked, congested, calcified, tight, or hardened
Aware and tingly, but not distractingly so	Too hot or cold
Connected with the spiritual world	Low self-esteem or timidity
Balanced interpersonal relationships	Vacated, dull, dark, or stagnant
In tune with personal power	Numb, without feeling, or distant
Clear perceptions and feelings	Pulsing with anxiety or fear
Control of incoming/outgoing chatter and energy	Throbbing uncomfortably
A mild, dense electrical current running through chakras	Systemically malfunctioning body/mind
The body's central core feeling is in alignment with the rest of the body	Invasive energy struggles
	Backaches or neck aches

As you read the preceding lists, think about times when you have noticed any of these indications of chakra activity. What was happening to you, and who were you with? What activity were you engaged in when you felt that you were sending or receiving energy-information? Recognizing these sensations is a good way to understand the language of your chakras and become more aware of how you intuitively interact with others. Next time you notice any of the chakra-language symptoms, stop and intuit the immediate interaction, thoughts, or situation. These symptoms are reminders that you are actively engaged in intuitive communication. Learn to notice and act on these messages, and you will reap the health benefits of a harmonious chakra system.

ARE YOU AWARE OF THE ENERGY-HEALTH OF YOUR CHAKRAS?

We do not know the real causes of illness. Doctors are treating the symptoms without knowing the cause.[19]

— Len Saputo, MD

Following are lists of activities that tend to affect the health and harmony of the chakra system. As you become better acquainted with the operation of your chakras, some of the things that have tended to deplete you will no longer do so. (See appendix 1 for more chakra health information.)

ACTIVITIES AND THINGS THAT...	
ENHANCE CHAKRA HEALTH	**DEPLETE CHAKRA HEALTH**
Creative expression	Absorbing another's pain or sadness
Speaking the truth	Deceit, lying, subterfuge, and competition
Practicing compassion and joyful living	Grounding through another person
Practicing being in the Now	Lack of energy protection and boundaries
Self-love and acceptance	Lack of grounding
Physical expressions: dance, yoga, sex, etc.	Fatalism, depression, and lethargy
Inspirational speakers, books, and movies	Some recreational and medicinal drugs
Self-healing and meditation	Power struggles
Healing and supporting others	Difficult relationship issues
Attention to physical and emotional well-being	Emotional or physical abuse
Listening to the body and spirit	Fear, pain, and anxiety
Positive thoughts	Negative thoughts

Think about the preceding lists of activities that directly affect the ongoing balance and vital energy available in your chakras. Do you engage in more "enhance" or "deplete" activities? Who tends to deplete or weaken your chakras? Who allows you to interact with them while maintaining your chakras in a vital state? Your intuitive awareness of this information will help you maintain the vitality of your chakras and allow you to choose a healthy lifestyle.

The following story illustrates how you can directly use chakra information in your healing meditations. It comes from a thirty-year-old woman who is a law firm administrator and a second-year Intuition Medicine practitioner:

Pulling a very black, ugly, even necrotic energy from my first chakra during a meditation, I discovered that it was from an ex-husband. It had attached to my chakra as a result of an injury he had inflicted on me that was causing major emotional, physical, and energetic blocks not only in my first chakra but throughout my entire energetic system (and manifesting physically and emotionally as well). When I cleared the black energy, I literally reexperienced the physical and emotional trauma from the injury. But during the meditation, I finally released all that ugly, stagnant energy. Within a week of pulling it out, my chiropractor was able to adjust my hip completely into place, and it held — which had never happened since my hip injury. Also, I regained the full range and ease of motion in my right hip, which I hadn't experienced in over twenty years. Years of old "stuff" released from me over the next several weeks.

My intention in this chapter has been to give you a humanistic working model for living with intuitive awareness of the subtle interactions among yourself, others, and the world around you. I trust that this chakra information will empower you to live in a healthy body.

Go to the next chapter, "The Chakra System Practice," when you feel ready for more introspective, daily-awareness, and healing practices.

Chapter 11

THE CHAKRA SYSTEM PRACTICE

The ancient Egyptian initiates understood the secret systems of spiritual culture whereby cosmic energy in man may be stimulated in the spinning vortices located along the spinal column and called chakras.

— Manley P. Hall

The focus of the chakra practice is to give you simple and powerful focus tools for locating, diagnosing, and healing your chakra system. This is a central component in practicing the Intuition Medicine model of self-healing, and it further strengthens your ability to use intuition as a human sense. If you are a beginning student, please do the chakra practice daily for about a month in order to integrate this new way of operating into your life. After that, a few times a week will maintain your development; more frequent practice will heighten your intuition.

Contemplative Meditations

There are two chakra meditations. The first is designed to guide you in locating and experiencing the energy of your chakras; it is a good one to practice for diagnostic purposes. The second adds the component of life-force and earth energy and is a chakra self-healing meditation. You may choose to do the two meditations one after the other or each alone.

Every so often, take time to reflect on your experiences with each of the chakra meditations. Follow the pre- and post-meditation questions after each of the meditations as a guide for further exploration; write notes on your personal reflections in your journal. Your chakras are your living library of knowledge — read and heal them often!

Observational Practices: Pre-Meditation Questions

Reflect on the following questions, and write your answers in your journal. Every so often, read your pre-meditation notes after a chakra meditation; see if you would revise any of your answers from a present-time perspective.

1. Which chakras are currently in an optimal state of harmony?

2. Which chakras are currently out of an optimal state of harmony?

Keep an ongoing list of the chakras that you find in harmony and those you find out of harmony. It is instructive to gauge your progress by occasionally looking at a longitudinal graph of your pattern of chakra health.

Chakra Grounding Meditation

• Place yourself in any comfortable meditation position.

• Bring your attention into your meditation sanctuary, and breathe slowly in through your nose and out through your mouth. Listen to the sound of your breath, and make this the most important thing you are doing right now. Breathe out any distraction and be present in your sanctuary. Keep listening to the sound of your breath. Do this focused breathing for one minute.

• Come into communication with yourself and sense the presence of yourself as spirit within your body. Perceive the energy of your spirit within your meditation sanctuary. Now affirm that your spirit energy is moving throughout your body and down into the ground, sending your spiritual roots into the earth. Be in your body, grounded to the earth. Affirm that your spirit is embracing your body. Hold that feeling for a moment.

- Dilate your feet chakras at the bottoms of your feet. Sense your feet anchoring into the earth. Affirm that your ankles, calves, knees, and thighs are grounding into the energy of the earth. Affirm that the energy in your pelvis and buttocks is dropping low to the ground. Affirm that your solar plexus and upper torso are relaxing and dropping into the grounding field of the earth. Now relax and ground your neck and shoulders. Drop the energy of your arms and hands low to the ground. Sense the energy of your neck, face, and head grounding into the earth. Now hold a whole-body sense of connecting as a spirit in your body to the gravity-grounding field of the earth. Hold that awareness for a moment.

- Now put your attention on your first chakra. Intuit an emotional-grounding symbol, and affirm that this symbol is an anchor pulling your energy down into the earth. Visualize your emotional energy flowing with the current of gravity and anchoring into the center of the earth. Feel the pull of gravity shifting your emotions to a low, slow frequency.

- Take a relaxing breath and center your attention in your meditation sanctuary. Scan your chakra system: seventh chakra at the top of your head; sixth chakra at your forehead; fifth chakra at your throat; fourth chakra at your sternum; third chakra at your solar plexus; second chakra at your navel; first chakra at the base of your spine; feet chakras at the soles of your feet; telepathic chakras around your eyes; and hand chakras in the palms of your hands.

- At your own pace, heal each of your chakras. Intuitively know which chakras are holding energy that is not in harmony with your sense of well-being. At each chakra, affirm "I am now grounding off all energy that is out of harmony with my well-being."

- End this meditation with deep, slow, relaxing breathing — in through your nose and out through your mouth. Come into communication with yourself as spirit. Greet yourself from the center of your meditation sanctuary. Affirm that your spirit is fully grounded into your body and chakras. Affirm that your spirit is grounding into the earth. Hold this intention to be fully grounded in body, mind, and spirit for one full minute.

Life-Force and Earth-Energy Meditation with the Chakras

In this second meditation, you will follow six steps with each chakra:

1. Visualize dilating the chakra.

2. Diagnose the energy in the chakra.

3. Ground off any aberrant current, images, colors, or sensations.

4. Fill the chakra with your life-force and earth energy.

5. Affirm a healing color, tone, symbol, or feeling in the chakra.

6. Calibrate the openness of the chakra to sustain health and harmony.

I recommended that you experiment with the openness setting — dialing up or down — of each chakra and do not have all chakras fully open. For most modern mystics, settings from 20 to 30 percent open work well for the first and second chakras. Set your third and fourth chakras according to your power and compassion needs. The fifth, sixth, hands, and feet chakras can be as open as is comfortable for you. Keep the seventh-chakra setting at 25 percent when you are "in the world" and more open during contemplative meditation. Set your telepathic chakras to your level of personal comfort. Use these general settings to begin with, as they work for most sensitive people. Experiment with a percentage of openness for each chakra; being too open or closed affects the healthy functioning of the chakra. Also see appendix 2 for more information on when to dial up and dial down your chakras.

Here is how to do this meditation:

- Place yourself in any comfortable meditation position.

- Drop your emotional energy low to the ground. Visualize a first-chakra grounding anchor. Hold that grounding field for a moment.

- Bring your attention into your meditation sanctuary, and breathe slowly in through your nose and out through your mouth. Listen to the sound of your breath, and make this the most important thing you are doing right now. Breathe out any distraction and be present in your sanctuary. Do this focused breathing for one minute.

- Go through your life-force and earth-energy meditation practice (see chapter 9).

- Open your first chakra and sense how it feels. Scan and notice areas of dark, congested, or murky energy, feelings, colors, or tones. Visualize your life-force energy running through the chakra and dissolving any unhealthy energy. Release the energy by running it down through your grounding connection and into the earth. Affirm a healing color, tone, symbol, or feeling in the chakra as you saturate it with life-force energy. Visualize setting the openness of this chakra for health. Breathe into this area and relax your lower back.

- Open your second chakra and sense how it feels. Scan the chakra and notice areas of dark, congested, or murky energy, feelings, colors, or tones. Visualize your life-force energy running through the chakra and dissolving any unhealthy energy. Release the energy by running it down through your grounding connection and into the earth. Affirm a healing color, tone, symbol, or feeling in the chakra as you saturate it with life-force energy. Visualize setting the openness of this chakra for health. Breathe into this area and relax your pelvis, back and front.

- Open your third chakra and sense how it feels. Scan and notice areas of dark, congested, or murky energy, feelings, colors, or tones. Visualize your life-force energy running through the chakra and dissolving any unhealthy energy. Release the energy by running it down through your grounding connection and into the earth. Affirm a healing color, tone, symbol, or feeling in the chakra as you saturate it with life-force energy. Visualize setting the openness of this chakra for health. Breathe into this area and relax your abdomen, back and front.

- Open your fourth chakra and sense how it feels. Scan and notice areas of dark, congested, or murky energy, feelings, colors, or tones. Visualize your life-force energy running through the chakra and dissolving any unhealthy energy. Release the energy by running it down through your grounding connection and into the earth. Affirm a healing color, tone, symbol, or feeling in the chakra as you saturate it with life-force energy. Visualize setting the openness of this chakra for health. Breathe into this area and relax your chest, back and front.

- Open your fifth chakra and sense how it feels. Scan and notice areas of dark, congested, or murky energy, feelings, colors, or tones. Visualize your life-force energy running through the chakra and dissolving any unhealthy energy. Release the energy by running it down through your grounding connection and into the earth. Affirm a healing color, tone, symbol, or feeling in the chakra as you saturate it with life-force energy. Visualize setting the openness of this chakra for health. Breathe into this area and relax your neck and shoulders, back and front.

- Open your sixth chakra and sense how it feels. Scan and notice areas of dark, congested, or murky energy, feelings, colors, or tones. Visualize your life-force energy running through the chakra and dissolving any unhealthy energy. Release the energy by running it down through your grounding connection and into the earth. Affirm a healing color, tone, symbol, or feeling in the chakra as you saturate it with life-force energy. Visualize setting the openness of this chakra for health. Breathe into this area and relax your forehead and face.

- Open your telepathic chakras and sense how they feel. Scan and notice areas of dark, congested, or murky energy, feelings, colors, or tones. Visualize your life-force energy running through the chakras and dissolving any unhealthy energy. Release the energy by running it down through your grounding connection and into the earth. Affirm a healing color, tone, symbol, or feeling in the chakras as you saturate them with life-force energy. Visualize setting the openness of the telepathic chakras for health. Breathe into this area and relax your eyes, nose, ears, and mouth.

- Open your seventh chakra and sense how it feels. Scan and notice areas of dark, congested, or murky energy, feelings, colors, or tones. Visualize your life-force energy running through the chakra and dissolving any unhealthy energy. Release the energy by running it down through your grounding connection and into the earth. Affirm a healing color, tone, symbol, or feeling in the chakra as you saturate it with life-force energy. Visualize setting the openness of this chakra for health. Breathe into this area and relax the top, back, and front of your head.

- Visualize your life-force energy running across your shoulders, down your arms, and into your open hand chakras. Saturate your hands with amplified currents of your healing energy. Then place your hands directly on any chakras that you intuit as needing more healing energy.

- Complete the chakra meditation by wrapping your arms around your body. Hold this position of self-love for a minute or more.

Observational Practices: Post-Meditation Questions

1. Make a copy of the Aura and Chakra Illustration for Diagnosis and Journaling on page 203 to use with this exercise. Gather crayons and colored pencils or pens for coloring and drawing.

Draw in the colors, symbols, and percentage of openness that you intuited in each chakra. Make notations of your observations.

2. Do you intuit that the colors, symbols, and percentage of openness you sensed will promote your optimal balance and health? If not, note the present highest healing color, symbol and percentage of openness for each chakra.

3. Look back at your answers to the pre-meditation questions. Did the information you received in the meditations change how you would answer them? If so, how?

4. Note how you received your information. Was it through images, sounds, words, feeling, symbols, colors, or knowing?

5. During the meditation, which chakras felt balanced?

6. Which chakras felt in need of attention?

7. Which chakras do you communicate from on a daily basis?

8. Which chakras do you tend to overlook or avoid?

9. Which chakras are most in need of your healing focus?

Daily-Living Tips

- Recognize when you are communicating from your chakras.

- Notice which chakras are your dominant senders and receivers.

- Notice which people and situations activate your chakras.

- Intentionally adjust your chakra settings for ease and comfort as you move through your day.

Experiments: Try This!

- Experiment with this if you are claustrophobic or simply do not like being in congested places, such as a crowded elevator or an airplane full of people. Dial down *all* your chakras to 10 percent, and you should feel very little or no energy coming in or going out. This tends to greatly lessen the feelings of being crowded by people. You can do this with your eyes open or closed.

- In a prone position on a bed, close your eyes and come into the Now in your meditation sanctuary. Put one of your hands on a chakra that is in need of healing and drop the other hand off the bed so that it points down toward the ground. Visualize the low hand making a grounding connection to the earth, inducing a siphon effect. Visualize the blocked or dis-eased energy in the chakra pulling out of the chakra and into the hand you have placed on the chakra. Visualize that energy immediately running up your arm, across your shoulders, down the opposite arm, and out your grounded hand into the earth. Continue to do this until you intuit a release of the dis-eased energy. Then, with your earth and life-force energies resonating through your body, place both hands on the same chakra and fill it up with your vital healing energy. Repeat until you intuit a harmony in the chakra.

Affirmations: Repeat Often

- I am abundant in my love of self and others.
- I practice compassion.
- I am expansive in my creative expression.
- I see goodness in myself and the world around me.
- I speak my lessons of wisdom.
- I practice truth.
- I am a modern mystic.

Trust

Your Intuition Medicine bag is in your hands and present with you now. Within your healing bag is this chakra formula: "I identify, interpret, and heal the energy of my chakras." Your medicine bag also holds this chakra prescription: "I intuitively perceive, trust, and follow through in my practice of chakra health."

Chapter 12
THE AURA: HALO OF LIGHT

The vital force is not enclosed in man but radiates within and around him like a luminous sphere. It may poison the essence of life and create disease, or it may purify and restore the health.

— Paracelsus

In our practice of Intuition Medicine, we refer to the field of energy around the body simply as the aura. Most people do not realize that they have a second skin — the aura is an energy skin that protects and shields their energy system just as physical skin protects their inner organs.

Imagine having no skin. What would happen? All your organs would spill out onto the ground. Your veins and arteries would sag and bulge. You would be defenseless against dirt, germs, and viruses. And, perhaps worst of all, you would look pretty frightening! Your skin is a highly efficient protective layer between you and the external world. It holds all of your organs in place, it shields you, and it filters out foreign matter that could be dangerous or irritating to your inner organs.

Like physical skin, the aura is permeated with natural disease-fighting chemistry, and it hosts the sensory communications of the nervous system. This second skin is the boundary between your personal energy system and the energy of your environment; an illuminated wrap of life-force medicine; and a subtle nervous system receiving and sending energy messages. This energy skin is your aura. Every living being has an aura.

177

The human aura field is distributed around the body like an ovoid, spherical, or egg-shaped cocoon of energy. Clairvoyantly, it appears as a shape with different qualities in different places. You may see the boundary as diffuse, well defined, smooth, or jagged (you may not see or feel the aura's separate, interior layers unless you focus your attention on them). You can perceive the aura clairvoyantly as color, brightness, darkness, shape, and density. You can hear the aura clairaudiently as tone, sound, music, frequency, and vibration. You can feel the aura using biotelemetry (the detection and measurement of a human or animal condition, activity, or function such as the heartbeat or body temperature) and psychometry (temperature changes, pulsation, tingling, pressure, or magnetism).

When you are feeling healthy, self-confident, calm, and grounded, your aura is healthy as well. A healthy aura is indicated by a cocoon of energy surrounding and extending out from the body at least one foot in all directions. This positive protection field is composed of bright colors, strong vibrations, pure tones, and a full, smooth, egg-shaped boundary. When you are sick, depressed, sad, or unsure of yourself, your aura is close to your body. The colors are most likely to be dull, murky, and dark. The frequency is slow and erratic. There may be breaks or tears in the boundary. And the shape could be bumpy and distorted. All of these indicate that your aura is not serving as a positive protection field between you and the energy of others and your environment.

An unprotective aura can be a cause of illness and distress for sensitive people. Without the natural filtering system of a positive protection field surrounding your body, you are open to environmental influences. The frequency of different energies can coexist and overlap nondestructively in the same space; take, for example, radio and television frequencies. Much of the energy in your environment — mental, physical, and emotional — may be positive, but much of it is negative.

THE HOLOGRAPHIC CORONA

Your aura acts as a reception and relay network for subtle energies. It delivers energy messages to the chakra system, which translates them into hormonal, nerve, and cellular activity in the physical body. In general, the aura tends to hold present (rather than past) thoughts, feelings, attitudes, and interactions between yourself and your environment. As the world first interconnects with your auric field, the freshest impressions, communications, and intuitive hits are woven into it. As an early-warning system, your aura also detects energy disturbance not yet manifested. This aspect of the aura's function is a preview of the future that can be utilized as a preventive tool.

Disease in the physical, emotional, or mental body is often preceded by a disturbance in the aura, or, if it originates within the physical body, it registers in the aura at the same time or oftentimes before it manifests in a person's conscious mind or physical body. I had a patient in the medical clinic years ago who was in good health and having her annual health checkup. The clinic doctor asked me to energetically scan her, and I picked up a reproductive-system problem in her aura. None of the medical tests confirmed my scan. Three weeks later she returned to the clinic because of uterine hemorrhaging. Your aura is an early-warning system for disease. By paying attention to such forewarnings, you can take preventive healing action, whether it is medical, psychological, or energetic.

A grounded aura allows you to sense when energy is being directed at you from near or far, and gives you the choice to accept it or cleanse it out of your space. This puts people and situations at a healthy distance from you, thus allowing them less power to unbalance you. With a grounded aura, you will feel safer and more secure, and the quality of all your grounding anchor points will improve. Your aura, when functioning effectively, acts as a lightning rod for negative energy or thoughts that enter your space. If your aura is not protecting you well, you might be hit by someone's unhealthy energy transference, or you might feel that you are being verbally attacked when someone is simply transmitting information. With a grounded aura, these undesirable intrusions into your system will be intercepted at the outer edge of your aura and automatically grounded out of your personal field and down into the earth. With practice, your aura will become an autonomic system of protection.

YOUR SPIRITUAL SKIN

The human aura is created by the action of life-force energy within the body as it resonates through the chakras and the physical and subtle anatomy. This life force radiates from the body, forming a cocoon of energy — the aura. This human corona is similar to an electromagnetic field radiating from an electrical device. Auras have been observed surrounding living systems from ancient times through contemporary investigations. Among those who work with the subtle-energy body, the aura is a universally accepted phenomenon.

Depictions of the aura can be found in the religious, mystical, and spiritual art and literature of almost every culture. It is often shown as a halo of light or circular symbol around the head or as a corona around the body. Symbolically, the luminous halo or corona signifies purity, saintliness, or enlightenment, and is a metaphor for spirituality. In particular, it may indicate a deity — a god or goddess. The aura indicates wisdom intelligence at work within the haloed person.

The Aura: A Universal Phenomenon

The Greek word *aura* means "breath" or "air." In many traditions, the terminology given to the human aura is synonymous or overlaps with the term used for life-force energy. Aura terminology from 1000 BC to the twenty-first century include a wide variety of names. In the traditions of early Hebrews, *ruach*; Hindus, *paramanu*; Cabalists, *yesod*; Hermetics, *telesma*; Gnostics, solar orb; Kabbalah mystics, *nefish*; Hawaiian Kahunas, *mana*; Christian Bible, golden bowl; and Christian mystics, aureole and nimbus. In the cultures of Germans, *wodan*; Peruvians, *huaca*; Sioux Indians, *wakan*; Eskimos, *sila*; Ituri Pygmies, *megbe*; Kalahari Bushmen, *rlun*; African Elgonyi, *ayik*; Pacific Ponape, *ani*; Congolese, *elima*; Australian Aborigines, *zogo*; Maoris, *atua*; and Yaqui, lines of the world. Philosophers and scientists from ancient to present times refer to the aura with different names: Plato, *nuos*; Erasistratus, *pneuma*; Paracelsus, *munia*; Blavatsky, astral light; Blondlot, N-rays; radiesthists, etheric force;

Gurwitsch, mitogenetic radiation; Grischenko, bioplasma; Puharich, psi plasma; de la Warr, prephysical energy; von Bertalanffy, anamorphosis; Worrall, paraelectricity; Muses, noetic energy; Burr, L-Field; and Tiller, magnetoelectricity.

In the field of energy medicine, *aura* is the most common name for this aspect of the subtle anatomy. Depending on the methodology, other names may be used to refer to the aura: astral body, biofield, biolumi-nescence, bioplasmic body, bioplasmic field, causal body, corona discharge, Divine rays, electric corona, electromagnetic body, energy body, etheric body, etheric web, golden web, health aura, intuitive body, Kirlian aura, light body, mental body, spiritual fire, spiritual skin, vitality sheath, web of frequency or web of light.

LAYERS OF LIGHT

All living matter, from a seed to a human being, is surrounded and controlled by electrodynamic fields.[1]

— Harold Burr

The aura is a seamless energetic skin with internal patterned layers or sheaths. These sheaths are like a *matryoshka* — a Russian nesting doll — as each layer surrounds another to form a whole (see the Aura Layers and Chakras illustration on page 182). Another visual metaphor is an onion, with a smooth exterior and a neatly arranged interior of concentric layers. The life-force energy emissions from the seven major chakras create the seven circular layers or sheaths of your aura.

The aura is an energetic weave of life force moving through the seven chakras. This electromagnetic action of the chakras generates seven distinct layers.

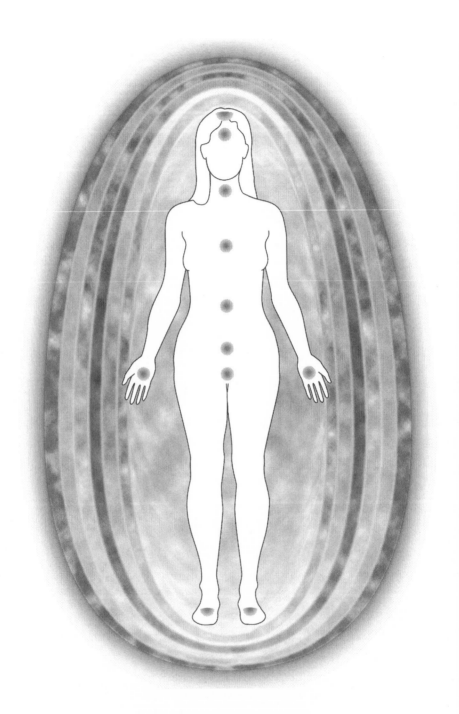

AURA LAYERS AND CHAKRAS

This auric web of light is distinct from the bioelectrical state of the physically based energy of the body. The entire energy body radiates with this spiritually based energy and pulses its currents around the physical body like sheaths of light that create your aura signature. An aura is like a signature piece of clothing — unique and individual.

In laboratory research, Dr. Valerie Hunt and Rosalyn Bruyere discovered that each color in a test subject's aura was associated with a different wave-pattern recorded at the seven chakra points on their skin. This confirmed the existence of the chakra system, as well as the extended subtle energies emitted by it. Those subtle energies were found to occupy an extended frequency range distributed around the body — the aura.[2] Measuring bodily radiations with electromagnetic detectors, Professor William Tiller plotted a seven-domain spectrum around the body. He described each domain as unique and able to carry several different radiations, not just one. I interpret this as the ability of the aura layers to hold multiple messages within each layer. As a metaphor, an email inbox holds many messages from different people together in one place. Tiller calls these fields "multiple auric sheaths around the body."[3]

The seven layers of the aura operate as antenna systems that relate to the seven chakras and the physical body via the endocrine glands. If there is a disturbance in a particular auric layer, a response to this disturbance will manifest in the physical body; when the disturbance originates in the physical body, a response will be mirrored in the aura. The ability to locate such a disturbance in either a particular layer of the aura or a specific body area is a useful diagnostic tool in the practice of energy medicine. This internal dowsing of body reactions opens an access window to information at subtle-energy levels, leading to enhanced intuition in both daily life and medical diagnostics.[4]

To further understand the function of the aura's layers, consider that biologists have measured the electromagnetic energy of each organ and system of the body as pulsing at a unique frequency, indicating that the body can function as a type of transmitting and receiving antenna. In this biological model, health is diagnosed (using the measurement tools of conventional medicine) as the body's electromagnetic field pulsing in coherence. A radio antenna can receive a range of frequencies; when the radio is tuned properly, it receives coherent radio broadcasts. The layers of your aura work in a similar way. With training, you can operate and control your auric antenna, improving your reception and transmission of energies.

THE SEVEN LAYERS OF THE AURA

A considerable number of consistent, reliable mystical and scientific reports provide evidence that layers of electromagnetic energy exist within the human aura. The seven layers of the aura generally correlate with the energies of the seven chakras, with some differences and additional functions. In this section, I describe the function of each auric layer, which you should visualize as a three-dimensional holograph, and provide additional information about that layer. I begin with the sheath of energy next to your physical body and move outward to the seventh layer, which is farthest away from your body, at the edge of your auric field.

The first auric layer, closest to the body, indicates the immediate health or disease of the physical body. For most people, this layer seems to be the easiest one to see and feel. This layer is the auric anchor to the physical earth, which metaphorically and literally shows the strength of the life force. When you are ungrounded or "out of your body," this layer is diffused or does not hug your skin. In people who are about to die, whether by accident or disease, I usually see this first layer as a dull, flat black, devoid of any pattern or movement. Conversely, I had a client who had a brilliant, full, sapphire-blue first layer, which I saw gave him great physical prowess. I later learned that he was an Olympic gymnast. A healthy first layer supports the vitality of the immune system as well.

The second layer of the aura flows concentrically and holographically around the first layer. This second layer is an emotional security blanket, wrapping the body with a feeling of safety and well-being. When this layer is healthy, your inner relationship with your sexuality is harmonious, which gives balance to your sexual expression with others. This is the layer where you display your feelings of attraction or rejection toward others — your energetic pheromone! When people are engaged in chaotic emotional or sexual relationships, this layer appears riddled with pebbled patterns or ripped lines. I once had a client who was happy in her profession as a prostitute; her second layer was radiant with a rainbow of pleasurable colors. Another client, who was experiencing an agonizing divorce, had bloody rips in her second layer, from her angry husband. A healthy second layer supports a balanced sexual identity and emotional body.

The third layer of the aura displays how you interface with your environment and society in general, as well as your expression of personal power in the world. A low pulse or diffuse layer shows a tentative, weak, or introverted interaction with the world. I often observe this layer as huge and gaily loud in performers, and delicate and pristinely quiet in monks and nuns. A healthy third layer shows a clear, purposeful attitude about yourself as a participant in your environment.

The fourth layer of the aura is where people display their hearts. It indicates whether they are humanitarians or Scrooges, beatific souls or miserly louses. This layer indicates the interactive emotions of your primary relationships with friends, partners, coworkers, and pets. Often the most recent interactions with others are held in living color in this layer. I once had a client who had an image of a crocodile in this layer; I was confounded until she spoke excitedly about having spent the morning at an aquarium, where she had been lovingly watching a pool full of crocodiles. Because auric layers often report that which is about to transpire, I have sometimes seen in this layer the images of an impending divorce. A healthy fourth layer embodies and develops a heart-centered, compassionate disposition.

The fifth layer of the aura indicates creative force and communication skills. This layer is a linking and transfer area, reflecting the transformation of spiritual perception and altruism into expressions of creativity and communication. Your satisfaction or disappointments with the creative forces in your life are displayed in this layer. When people are happy with their career choices, this is an ebullient and buoyant layer; those who are languishing in a boring occupation often have a sandpaper pattern, dull colors, and slow movement of energy through this layer. I have observed stellar speakers rainbowed with a glowing, burnished fifth layer while giving presentations. Conversely, timid people and those who do not trust their creative force have quite narrow bands of energy in this layer. A healthy fifth layer contributes to embodied inspiration.

The sixth layer of the aura is the immediate depiction of intuitive development and intelligence. This layer shows the development of the doorway to the subtle realms of the world — the mystic's portal to what most people call the unseen world. When this mystical sense is integrated, the sixth layer is broad and full of light. Those who perceive the world from a linear and analytical viewpoint, on the other hand, have a small, brittle-patterned layer. A convicted felon who I observed in a police lineup had a shriveled, black sixth layer. I had the privilege of studying with a Hindu master who had a crystalline, diamond-blue sixth layer. A healthy sixth layer supports heightened intuitive perception and respect for life.

The seventh layer of the aura is the cloth woven of your spirituality. Spirituality is your connection to God, Goddess, the Divine — whatever that means to you. Highly developed, evolved individuals radiate a notable light in this layer, an almost ethereal glow. This layer, coupled with the sixth layer, is what most people see around the head and describe as the "halo of light" or "corona of color." Most young children have the light of this spiritual glow from birth, but unfortunately it diminishes with immersion in the physical and mental world. Your aura glow and your connection to the Divine can be cultivated and strengthened by filling this layer with your spiritual light. As the Bible says, "If thine eye be single, thy whole body will be filled with light."[5]

SENSING THE AURA

How do we see physically? No different than we do in our consciousness — by means of the productive power of imagination. Consciousness is the eye and ear, the sense for inner and outer meaning.[6]

— Novalis

A comment I often hear in aura training is "I do not see layers." Most students do perceive energy around the head, though, and some emanation of color, sound, pulse, or pattern within the aura. Often, the strongest chakra energy creates the dominant or "loudest-resonance" layer in the aura, and the other layers operate at a subtler, quieter level. For example, if someone is angry, you may see only a red aura. If a person is ill, you may see primarily a dull, gray field of energy.

The aura's light is subtle to most Western eyes; clairvoyance requires stimulation in order to train the inner eye to perceive the subtle light-energy of the aura. When you perceive clairvoyantly, you are setting ocular vision aside and engaging the inner eye to see subtle energy. Besides an outer light and eyes, sight requires an "inner light," one whose luminescence complements the familiar outer light and transforms raw sensation into meaningful perception. You can stimulate your ability to see the entire panoply of the aura's layers (and other subtle-energy fields) through the use of hand psychometry. Psychometry involves meridian connections into the pineal gland, which stimulates the light-sensitive clairvoyant perception. Whether or not you feel energy in your hands, moving your hands in front of your chakras and through your aura stimulates currents of signal energy, which travel up your arms and into your pineal gland. This energy pathway tweaks the light-sensitive pineal gland to function at a higher level in perceiving subtle variations of light. With practice, your ability to perceive your aura's light and layers will improve. My observation of a connection between the hands (psychometry) and clairvoyance (the sixth chakra and corresponding pineal gland) directed me to research conducted by Dr. Fritz-Albert Popp, who in 1973 built the first photon detector sensitive enough to study biophotons. Based on his study of a hand-to-head bioenergy connection, I emailed him an inquiry asking if there exists a measurable photon-emission correlation between the hands and forehead, and, if so, whether the emissions are carried by a biophoton pathway. My assumptions were confirmed as correct in a recent email from Dr. Popp's office.

Numerous intuitives report feeling palpable sensations when they move their hands close to, but do not touch, the body. Normally these sensations are symmetrical, smooth, and evenly distributed around the body. However, different intuitives may experience different sensations when moving their hands around the body of the same individual. If illness or injury is present, a distinct sensation is noted near that part of the body. This may be experienced as heat, coolness, tingling, stickiness, or other feelings in the hands. Make it part of your journal practice to write down the sensations you feel and to draw the images you perceive when scanning your own aura; this will contribute immensely to the development of your intuition vocabulary. Whatever you experience is your personal language of intuition; that language will build upon itself as you acquire intuitive wisdom.

A twenty-two-year-old university student and first-year Intuition Medicine practitioner felt her life change as she became acquainted with her aura:

> *When I started consciously working on my aura, I could only imagine and trust that it was there based on what I had heard from others. Now I can see my aura and feel a pressure and temperature change as it strengthens. Creating a stronger aura has given me a sense of freedom. I can get more important things done without other people's agendas popping into my head constantly. My aura boundary has also given me a deepened appreciation that my daughter and husband have all they need on their paths without my interference.*

PERSPECTIVES ON THE AURIC FIELD

The colors in our aura reflect the character of our soul.[7]

— Edgar Cayce

The layers of the aura are a template and matrix of health and disease. Scanning each of the seven layers of your aura gives you a current health evaluation and diagnosis. When you become expert at scanning or simply maintaining your aura at optimal health, you will be able to discover most disease before it becomes a physical or psychological issue. Many, if not all, dissonant emotions can be cleansed from your auric field before you absorb their ill effects. In this manner, your aura acts as an early-warning system.

Another key function of the aura is to absorb and contain life-giving energy. Imagine your aura as a solar panel; when charged with light, it supplies vital force through all your systems; when depleted, all systems operate below normal health or cease to function well.

Your aura acts as a multipurpose broadcast system, much like a broadband radio; it sends out your energy and messages and receives messages, thoughts, emotions, and energy from the world. Your aura can hold these energy messages like an email inbox, but leaving them unanswered can cause an overload of dissonant frequencies to mix with your life-force energy. This mixing of frequencies can cause discomfort: voices in your head, ceaseless mental conversation, feeling crowded or claustrophobic, or a sense of lacking personal space. I suggest that you read and answer or delete your aura-energy messages daily. As you become more practiced at recognizing the incoming and outgoing energy fluctuations in your aura, you will be able to immediately respond to these energy messages, thereby maintaining the health and integrity of your aura energy.

The outer edge of your aura functions as your emotional boundary and psychic protection; this is your energy epidermis. Indeed, when this function is weak or lacking, the outer world merges and mixes with you, and your uniqueness is compromised by this blending of energies. The best of the world's love, joy, and happiness may merge with your own energy and inspire you or make you feel better, but your aura cannot sustain the energy of others without lowering its personal health frequency. People often intentionally allow energies from other people to blend with their own because they lack self-love, or they are afraid to take responsibility for their personal power, or they believe that the answer is outside themselves. This merging with other people's energy creates an aura of lowered vitality that is an energetic cause of illness.

THE ELECTRIC BODY OF HEALTH

The superior physician cures before the illness is manifested. The inferior physician can only care for the illness which he was unable to prevent.[8]

— Chinese aphorism

You are enmeshed in an ebb and flow of energy exchange with everyone and everything around you. Every living organism is born, lives, and dies in a sea of electromagnetic radiation, and all of life has evolved in an environment consisting of electromagnetic energy. As a result, the interactions that take place between living organisms and electromagnetic energy are crucial to life. To deny these interactions would be to deny the fundamental interaction upon which every living thing on the planet depends. The pulsing magnetic fields of the earth, cosmos, machines, and creatures all affect the energy field of your aura and, in turn, your body, mind, and spirit.[9]

The acupuncture practice of Chinese medicine deals with the invisible levels of energy. A skilled acupuncturist reads the pulses of the physical body to determine whether there is an imbalance in the counterpart of the energy body. The physician then rebalances the energy flow to prevent physical or mental disease. A noteworthy piece of history: in ancient China, patients paid doctors to keep them from getting sick. If they did fall ill, the doctors paid them. In Russia, acupuncture is used as an adjunct to psychotherapy.

Your aura is the mirror of your health and life. Like film imprinted with a light-produced image, your aura registers the intentions of your thoughts, moods, and actions. A living communication system, your aura sends information to the world around you and receives information from it.

A thirty-year-old second-year Intuition Medicine practitioner had a dramatic experience when expanding his aura. At 5 feet tall and 120 pounds, he is a small-statured Cirque du Soleil performer, but he has a huge, charismatic aura. Here is his aura story:

In 2002, I was meditating before a show for the NBA Sacramento Kings'
opening season. I set my intention to expand my aura to touch the capac-
ity crowd of fans in Arco Arena. After the show, the promoters told me
that they had never seen anything transpire between an audience and a
performer like they had just witnessed. All the fans in the stadium were
silent during my act, and when I took my final bow at the end, the
silence broke into screaming pandemonium. I couldn't believe that I had
expanded my aura; I really did feel like I touched all of the 17,613 fans in
the audience.

A PRACTICAL PROTECTION AURA IN DAILY LIFE

Is it possible that there exist human emanations which are still unknown to
us? Do you remember how electric currents and "unseen waves" were
laughed at? The knowledge about man is still in its infancy.[10]

— Albert Einstein

A highly healthy aura nourishes us with a constant circulation of life
force. It also protects us, because a high-energy fields disintegrate energy
that enters from lower-energy fields.

In order for your aura to act as positive protection and illuminated
healing energy, it must be in a whole and healthy state of coherence.
When your aura is filled with life force, others will show respect for your
boundaries. With a diagnostic scan, you can locate and heal aberrations
in the field of your aura. With intention and affirmation, you can quickly
revive the potent vitality of your aura's protective qualities. You need not
be in quiet meditation to practice aura diagnosis and healing; they can
and should be part of your practical daily awareness.

When you leave your home, the best health initiative is to walk into
the outside world with a grounded, vibrant aura. Physical, mental, or
emotional abuse of any kind — real or imagined; from within yourself
or from your environment — can affect all of your subtle-energy systems

when you are not being conscious. At times, your positive intentions may be pushed out of focus, and you may find yourself unprotected and affected by chaos from the world or ill intentions from other people. These are the times to be energetically proactive. Immediately scan your aura for aberrant patterns — energies that are not yours and have attached themselves to your auric field and are operating below your level of positive intention.

The following story illustrates how to actively work with your aura in daily life. It comes from a twenty-five-year-old corporate secretary who is a highly clairsentient second-year Intuition Medicine practitioner. She had difficulty with a boss who constantly intimidated her; she felt his energy pushing out her own feelings and thoughts, leaving her speechless and vulnerable in his presence. She described this situation as a "violation of boundaries," but she has now learned to use her aura as positive protection during these episodes.

> *The biggest aura revelation for me was discovering that the ways in which I had always tried to protect myself (being defensive, withdrawn, shut down, and angry) were energy drains in and of themselves, and that my boss was still able to "get in" and drain my energy. The discovery of being grounded, being aware of my auric field (which I think was probably very diminished back then), keeping my auric field grounded, and having healthy energy circulating through my aura literally changed my experience of life. Now I truly feel safe and protected, and I am almost immediately aware when someone or something is trying to violate my boundaries — or if I'm ungrounded, energetically unprotected, or vulnerable. I feel like a different person than I was a year ago.*

Here is how to create an aura of positive protection: First, affirm or visualize that your aura is entirely surrounding you and is grounded into the earth. You can clairvoyantly or clairsentiently scan for leaks in your aura; holes or tears indicate that someone is angry at or envious of you, and streaks of energy that are not of your aura's color or pattern indicate invasive mental messages. If you leave home feeling bright and happy, then find yourself feeling upset or gloomy without apparent cause, this can indicate a lack of aura boundary or body grounding, or perhaps that your attention is out of your body and not centered in your meditation sanctuary. You can test for this by scanning the shape of your aura and sensing whether it is equally full all around your body; where you lack an expansive energy skin, your body is unprotected. For example, if your aura is closer to you in back and farther out in front, you are more likely to get backaches or neck aches; if your aura is diminished at your legs and feet, you will tend to have cold feet. The strength and fullness of your aura protects your body and continually bathes it in healing life force; a lack of this constant state of healing provides an entry for dis-ease. Do not leave home without a vibrant, healthy cocoon of light surrounding you. Your aura is your body halo. Your aura is your protective energy skin; when it is compromised, you will often compensate with other ways to protect yourself.

A thirty-year-old high-school teacher and first-year Intuition Medicine practitioner often felt the angst and anger of her teenage students:

> *Before I learned how to create my aura as a protective field, I would clench my muscles as protection from unwanted energy when I felt that I was "under attack" from my students. Now, when I revert to clenching parts of my body, I know that my aura needs work. I cannot express how wonderful it is to sit within a self-made bubble of protection with the feeling of no one else being present in my space.*

Aura Protection Images

Play with some of the following aura protection visualizations and see what works for you. Change the images when you are in different situations during your day.

• A golden net

• An arboretum

• A clear crystal sphere

- A rainbow of light
- Spinning discs
- Silver swords
- A nurturing womb
- Sounds — bells, drums, chants
- A forest of grounded trees
- A moss-covered rock
- Symbols of love, compassion, and altruism
- A luminescent white pearl
- Gems and minerals
- A mirror
- A translucent bubble (like Glinda the Good Witch in *The Wizard of Oz*)
- A waterfall

AURA MEDITATIONS

To heal means to release obstruction (demons, germs, despair) between the sickness and the force of life driving towards wholeness.[11]

— Robert Becker

Positive energy nourishes and heals your body, mind, and spirit, and this is done most potently through meditation practice. Aura meditation (see the next chapter) can boost your overall health. A morning aura meditation seeds the rest of your day with the power of your positive intentions. You can set a specific goal for the day and quietly repeat that intention several times during the day, continuing to nourish and ground your energy. Your evening aura meditation cleanses and closes your day. It is a peaceful retrospective on the day's lessons and discoveries.

There is a direct correlation between a vibrant aura and good health. Without a daily dose of aura meditation, a sensitive person can quickly become unwell. The following story illustrates this point. It comes from a twenty-year-old hairstylist and second-year practitioner of Intuition Medicine who worked in a beauty salon with her boyfriend and his previous girlfriend. She found herself in a triangle of jealousy and competition, which made her ill when she forgot to practice her Intuition Medicine.

After about a month of not practicing my usual daily aura meditation, I became ill. In meditation, I noticed almost immediately that my aura was collapsed on all sides. Unfortunately, I did not do energy healing right away, but rather I went through the illness as a purely physical experience (perhaps I needed to learn something). I noticed that when my aura was down, I palpably felt the presence of my boyfriend's ex-girlfriend in my space. I felt that I had no protection. I felt like she was attempting to energetically merge into my aura to feel what was going on in my relationship with her ex-boyfriend. I found myself highly fearful, which is not a normal circumstance. I also felt as though a foreign energy overlaid my entire body like a net. When I began to cleanse my aura, the fear subsided as well as the feeling that I was being invaded by her jealous, negative energy. Since this episode, I have felt that I am better at visualizing and clearing my aura, and I now make time each morning to meditate.

ARE YOU PRACTICING AURA AWARENESS?

The universe seen from within is light; seen from without, by spiritual perception, it is thought.[12]

— Rudolf Steiner

When you first start working with your aura and noticing how you operate in the world, you may see your aura as a defense mechanism.

As your practice continues, you will realize that there is much more to the function of your aura than protection. With a healthy aura, you are more fully present and supportive for others. In maintaining your own aura integrity, you are a witness for others, allowing them to experience the full range of their own emotions and reactions without outside interference or judgment. This way of operating in the world allows you to hold the integrity of your own space and to honor yourself and others.

Here is an observation from a thirty-three-year-old Registered Nurse and third-year Intuition Medicine practitioner:

As a nurse, I thought the best way to support and facilitate healing in others was to give away my energy to those who needed it more than I did. Since I was strong and happy, I thought I could share those gifts. Unfortunately, working this way left me depleted and hollow; it wasn't until I studied auras that I became aware of the necessity of energy boundaries and how my aura could protect me. I now know that I can help someone without falling completely into their world, without feeling their pain and suffering. Now I allow people to experience their process of healing, and I support them without joining them in that experience.

HEALTHY AURA, HEALTHY BODY

Your physical sensations are a good indication of the state of your aura. Are you feeling vibrant, energized, and strong, or are you feeling lethargic, dull, and weak? The goal of Intuition Medicine is to help you move toward a vibrant self. As you learn to maintain your aura in a state of positive protection, you will find yourself feeling more consistently upbeat, self-confident, and healthy.

Take a moment to look at the following lists, and see how many of the "in harmony" and "out of harmony" descriptions are part of your experience. You can quickly diagnose the strength or weakness of your aura by comparing your feelings with the "in" and "out" lists.

HOW IT FEELS WHEN YOUR AURA IS...

IN HARMONY	OUT OF HARMONY
Connected to inner self and spirit	Neglectful of self and spirit
Connected to others without merging	Engaged in unhealthy lifestyle choices
Full of self-love	Not healing yourself when you need it
More present in your meditation sanctuary	Easily distracted; not present
Able to live authentically	Vulnerable, unsure, or afraid
Chakras in harmony	Defensive or reactive
Enclosed, protected, and secure	Responding inappropriately
Full of your own energy	Having difficulty containing feelings
Healthy emotional boundaries	Feeling unwanted energies in your space
Expansive, safe, and loving with others	Losing yourself in interactions with others
Confident, friendly, and cheerful	Easily invaded, judged, or not seen
Less internally defensive	Feeling exposed or raw
Complete; full of self	Primarily focused on protection
Harmonic, vibrant, and alive	Drained by any interaction with others
Clothed, protected, and comfortable inside your body	Tired, grumpy or withdrawn
Like a warm security blanket	Needing to be alone; needing rest to rejuvenate
Able to sense a clear inner voice	Anxious when interacting with others
Able to sense someone staring at you	Clenching muscles as a defensive gesture
Able to tell when someone is behind you	Feeling fearful anticipation without cause
Not anxious or agitated in crowds	Exposed, vulnerable, or porous
Able to say no with ease and without guilt	Feeling pain or discomfort from the environment
Able to sense a subtle extension of skin nerve endings	Experiencing jolts of feelings unrelated to circumstances
Able to be in a situation that previously diminished your grounding	Feeling scattered energy; "forward" and in your head
Receiving respectful communication from others	Vulnerable, unsure, or tentative
	Unable to detect bad circumstances
	Feeling discomfort when energies enter your space

It is a good practice to identify a couple of symptoms that indicate to you whether your aura is operating as a protective boundary; these indicators can become part of your intuition toolbox. For example, you know that your aura is healthy when you feel your own energy strongly and you connect to others without depletion or merging; you feel appreciation and respect for other people. A converse example would be when you feel vulnerable, unsure, and smothered or crowded by others; you get irritated easily, and you react like a mother bear to aggressively defend your space.

Take a moment to read and reflect on these questions:

- Think about times when you have felt or seen your aura. What were the sensations of your aura awareness at those times?

- Think about times when you intuitively perceived another person's aura. How did you perceive the aura — through clairvoyance, clairsentience, knowing, or another method?

Using your aura perceptions as an intuitive language, you can become more aware of subtle communication when you interact with others. The next time you perceive another person's aura — even slightly — stop and interpret the relationship of the energy perception to the immediate interaction, thoughts, or situation you are involved in. Learn to notice and act on these intuitive messages; they are your universal human language.

ARE YOU AWARE OF YOUR AURA HEALTH NEEDS?

Use the light within you to regain your natural clearness of sight.[13]

— Lao-tzu

Lists of activities and things that tend to affect the health and harmony of the aura follow on the next page. You might agree or disagree with the entries; feel free to add your own entries to these lists. As you become more aware of your aura's role as both a protection boundary and a cocoon of health energy, some of the things that tend to deplete you will no longer do so.

YOUR AURA AS BOUNDARY AND HEALING PROTECTION IS...	
ENHANCED BY...	**DEPLETED BY...**
Daily meditation and grounding practice	Neglecting daily meditation practice
A nurturing home space	Not paying attention to yourself
A harmonious work environment	Overworking or over thinking
Self-love, affirmations, and strong grounding	Long sedentary times; not moving enough
Exercise and nature walks	Verbal, physical, or energy attacks
Being with healthy people and animals	Interacting with negative people
Taking care of your body's needs	Worry, mental obsession, and fear
A nutritious diet	Constant thoughts about the future
Good thoughts; a positive outlook	Noise
Consciously intending an aura of light	Being exposed to media-communicated violence
Conscious breathing	Depressing thoughts; unclear intentions
Acts of kindness	Electrical devices: computers, TV, and radio
Singing, laughing, and smiling	Crowds of people
Speaking the truth	Not speaking the truth
Respecting yourself and others	A constant focus on negativity
Admiring beauty	Compulsive caretaking of others
Trusting your intuition	Not trusting your intuition
Being fully present as a spirit in your body	Neglecting necessary boundaries
Being present in the world	Merging with others' pain, worry, or grief
Living in a state of grace	

Reflect on the preceding lists; do you engage in more of the "enhance" or "deplete" activities? Who do you intuit to be the people in your life with vibrant auras, and how do these people affect you? Who do you intuit as having weak auras, and how are you affected by these people?

Health is a choice; as you read this book, you are gaining more practical knowledge about making wise choices in creating your body of health.

I hope that this chapter has given you insight into the experience of your own aura and how you can use your auric field as a vibrant cocoon of healing energy, a protective skin, and a passport to walking through the world with ease and grace.

Go to the next chapter, "The Aura Meditation and Healing Practice," when you feel ready to learn how to use your aura as a health tool, as positive protection, and as a source of boundary grounding. The time you spend in aura practice, even if it is five minutes a day, will give you immediate health benefits.

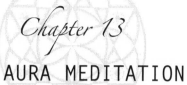

Chapter 13
THE AURA MEDITATION
AND HEALING PRACTICE

A magnetic field radiates from man... but this is not as physical substance,
but is as ethereal spirit, pure living, which pervades all things.

— J.B. von Helmont

$\mathcal{T}$he aura practice simply and powerfully enables you to perceive, diagnose, and heal your aura. This further strengthens your ability to use intuition as a human sense. You may need practiced repetition to fully sustain your abilities.

Contemplative Meditations

Two practices are presented here. The aura healing meditation is designed to guide you in perceiving and experiencing the energy of your aura as a protective cocoon and psychic boundary. This meditation strengthens, protects, and establishes boundaries.

The second practice is an aura healing procedure and includes a diagnostic process. This more formal, technical project works well with repetition as a way to continually fine-tune your intuitive skills. This is an explorative project that will continually update your information on the health of your aura.

You may choose to do the two practices one after the other or to just to do one at a time. I suggest that you record your answers to the pre-meditation questions in your journal before you do either the meditation or healing practice. Afterward, take time to reflect on your experiences with the aura meditation and healing practice and read the post-meditation questions. After doing both practices, write notes on your personal reflections in your journal as a guide for further exploration.

Observational Practices: Pre-Meditation Questions

1. How does your aura feel right now?

2. Intuit times or activities that help you maintain a strong protective aura.

3. Intuit times or activities that deplete the protective ability of your aura.

4. Make copies of the Aura and Chakra illustration on the following page so that you have blank charts for future use. On one copy draw the colors, symbols, patterns, and shape of your aura. Date each aura drawing.

Aura Healing Meditation

- Close your eyes and bring your attention into your head; find your quiet, still meditation sanctuary and be there.

- Greet yourself and listen to your inner voice.

- With focused breath, bring air in through your nose and exhale through your mouth. Continue to breathe in this way for one minute. Focus on your breath and release all other thoughts.

- Drop your energy and emotions low to the ground. Sense the force of gravity pulling your body to the center of the earth. Hold this feeling for a moment.

- With feeling and intention, visualize the energy at your lower back and the base of your spine dropping into the pull of gravity.

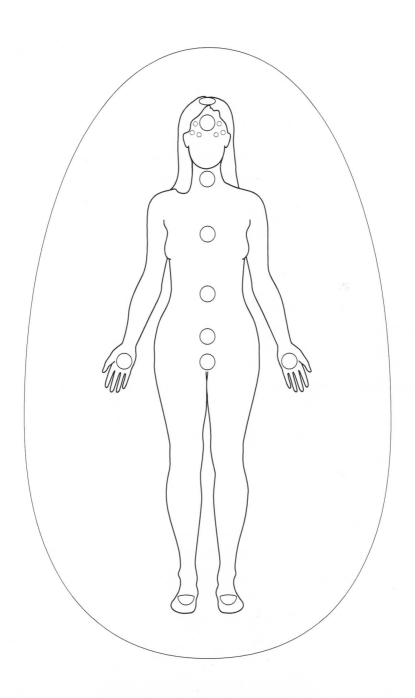

**AURA AND CHAKRA ILLUSTRATION
FOR DIAGNOSIS AND JOURNALING**

Now feel the energy throughout your body dropping low to the ground and flowing into the pull of gravity.

- With your attention in your meditation sanctuary, affirm that you would like to see and know a symbol that represents your emotional grounding. Trust the first knowing and insight you receive. Use this emotional-grounding symbol and visualize it anchoring your body into the core of the earth.

- Sense yourself dropping your emotional-grounding anchor symbol deep into the earth. Hold that feeling for a minute.

- Expand this feeling of your grounding as wide as your aura. Hold this setting for a moment.

- Open your feet chakras and feel the pulse of the electromagnetic current below your feet. Visualize pulling this earth energy up through your feet. Direct this earth energy up your legs to your first chakra, then drop the energy through your emotional grounding and back into the earth.

- Meditate on this circular flow of earth energy for a moment. Imagine your body being bathed in this magnetic healing current. Hold that feeling for a moment.

- From your meditation sanctuary, trust your intuition and affirm that you are sensing a symbol, color, or tone that represents your life-force healing energy. Trust the first information that comes to you.

- Visualize placing your life-force healing symbol above yourself within the top of your aura. Visualize this symbol generating life-force energy throughout your aura, showering from the top of your aura and flowing around and through your auric cocoon.

- Sense a cocoon of healing light and energy equidistant around your body. Hold that feeling for a moment.

- Intuit a personal protection symbol, color, or sound and visualize or affirm placing that protection symbol all around the outside perimeter of your aura. (Imagine that the perimeter of your aura is like the shell of an egg.) Ground that protection field into the earth.

- Repeat the Affirmations for the Seven Layers of the Aura, found at the end of this chapter.

- Direct your life-force energy through your aura, and run the current down through your grounding field with the intention of anchoring your whole aura into the earth.

- Hold that meditation setting for a quiet minute or more.

The Aura Diagnosis and Healing Practice

This is a fun and interesting experiment that gives you a great deal of information in each session. Play with this hands-on project to activate and fine-tune your intuitive sense. The best approach is to have an open, objective mind with no expectations of outcome. The directions are long, so I suggest you read them through completely before you begin.

Start by sitting in a quiet place with your eyes closed and being in your meditation sanctuary. Follow this preparation protocol, and then establish the integrity of your energy by following these steps:

- Hold your perception in your meditation sanctuary, for clear intuitive perception; keep your energy field grounded in present time.

- Visualize your personal protection symbol around the outside perimeter of your aura to maintain energy boundaries.

- Set an intention to facilitate the energy healing from your highest level of integrity for the greater good of yourself.

Aura Healing Protocal

The step-by-step protocol for aura diagnosis and healing follows.

1. Review the definition of the aura layers on the following page.

2. Diagnose the aura.

3. Heal the aura using life-force and earth energy.

4. End with a closure meditation.

The Aura's Seven Layers

This list is a helpful summary of the functions of the seven layers.

THE AURA'S SEVEN LAYERS		
LAYER	**REPRESENTS**	**DEALS WITH**
1st	Health	Physical being; grounding
2nd	Emotions	Feelings of well-being, relationships, and sexual identity
3rd	Personal power	The image you hold of yourself; worldly interactions
4th	Love	Love concepts, compassion, humanitarianism, and relationships
5th	Creativity	Expression in career; actualization of self in the world
6th	Visions	Intuitions, hopes, and the future
7th	Spiritual identity	Knowing the self; personal spirituality; protection

Diagnose the Energy of the Aura

In this step, use hand psychometry, along with your other intuitive skills, to scan and detect the condition of the auric field. Visualize this field of energy as a cocoon surrounding the body. Look at each layer of the aura, noting the following characteristics:

- Fullness or lack of energy.

- Brightness, amplitude, and amperage (the strength of an energy current).

- Temperature, vibration, and resonance.

- Degree of boundary and protection provided by the perimeter layer.

- Texture, pattern, weave, frequency, sound, color, symbol, and messages.

This procedure will give you a map to follow during the next step, healing the aura.

Do the Energy Healing Work

Use visualization or your hands to direct the healing life-force and earth energy into your aura.

- Fill in holes, tears, or spaces devoid of energy with life force.

- Create a coherence of temperature, sound, and pulse.

Bring Closure to the Healing Session

Complete the healing session with these two visualizations:

- Visualize a symbol, color, or tone to act as a perimeter boundary.

- Visualize grounding the aura in the Now.

Observational Practices: Post-Meditation Questions

If you wish, write notes and reflections in your journal in response to the following questions. It is always best to do journaling immediately following your meditations and healings.

1. Write a general list of observations regarding your perception of your aura.

2. How do you sense your aura: through clairvoyance, clairsentience, psychometry, knowing, or another method?

3. Do you perceive colors, patterns, sounds, frequencies, temperature, amplitude, density, or symbols in your aura?

4. Do you perceive a protective boundary between yourself and the world?

5. Do you perceive a vibrant health resonance in your aura?

6. Are areas of your aura in need of strengthening?

7. Using the illustration on page 203, draw the colors, symbols, patterns, and shape of your aura once again. Date each drawing.

8. Every so often, look at your pre- and post-meditation aura drawings longitudinally. This is very instructive in gauging your healing progress.

Daily-Living Tips

*   Begin to notice the state of your aura throughout the day. Be aware of times when it is functioning as a positive protective shield. Sense when it is allowing other people's energy to enter your personal space.

*   Several times during the day, take a few minutes to clear and upgrade the health of your aura. From the center of your meditation sanctuary, perceive the energy around your body and sense how far your aura extends. Sense the energy in the back, sides, and front of your auric-energy skin. Affirm that a healing waterfall of life-force energy is showering through your aura. Affirm that the energy of your aura is flowing down into the grounding field of the earth.

*   Several times during the day, take a few minutes to establish a grounded auric protection field. Affirm that a protective energy surrounds the outside of your aura, and electrically ground it deep into the core of the earth.

Experiments: Try This!

*   Have you ever been in a roomful of people and seen a person walk in and all heads turn to look at him or her? I see this as a manifestation of the person's aura filling up the room, reaching out and touching people like an energy handshake. Others call this charisma. If you would like to bring attention to yourself during a speech, in a group, or for whatever reason, try this with your aura: After you are grounded, fill your aura with bright colors and

expand your auric field into a large, grounded cocoon around your body. Experiment first at home to find out how much you can expand your aura and which size is comfortable for you. Some people can fill an entire room with their aura and feel comfortable and grounded, while others become scattered when their auras are expansive.

- If you would like to not be noticed, try this with your aura: After you are grounded, fill your aura with a soft or quiet color, then shrink your aura tightly around your body. To my amusement, when I do this, people who know me often ask if I have lost weight or tell me they thought I was much taller!

- Try this with another person: Have one person sit in a chair and ground her or his aura and then fill it with bright colors. Have the seated person intuitively sense the configuration and boundary of his or her aura but does not tell this information to the other person until after he or she has completed the experiment. The second person stands about four or more feet in front of the seated person, with both hands raised to chest height and palms facing the seated person. The standing person walks slowly toward the seated person with hands raised until s/he senses the edge of the seated person's aura. The standing person should remain at the perimeter of the seated person's field (not going into the auric field), then ask if this is where the seated person experiences or visualizes the edge of his or her aura. Next, the standing person walks around the entire perimeter of the seated person's aura and maps its outer edge from top to bottom. Upon returning to the front of the seated person, the standing person holds her or his hands at the aura perimeter and asks the seated person to visualize pulling his or her aura close to the body. Discuss what you both experience.

Affirmations for the Seven Layers of the Aura: Repeat Often

Repeat these seven affirmations as healing words for each layer of your aura. When affirmed together, they create a whole-aura healing.

- 1st   My body is an extension of the regenerative power of nature.

- 2nd   I feel the world as a dynamic source of enriching experiences.

- 3rd   I actively expand my will to explore the limitless realms of inspiration.

- 4th   I am a continual source of self-nourishing love.

- 5th   Listening to my inner voice, I create with ease and enjoyment.

- 6th   I clearly see the infinite abundance of the universe.

- 7th   I powerfully and positively create my own reality.

Trust

As you walk along the lifelong path of intuitive wisdom, hold your head up and remember to bask in the rays of the sun and to notice the beauty and magic of the moon and the stars. Walk through this life with ease and grace, and allow others to do the same.

Chapter 14
COLOR: THE LANGUAGE OF ENERGY

Mere color, unspoiled by meaning and unallied with definite form, can speak to the soul in a thousand different ways.

— Oscar Wilde

You have a visceral, emotive relationship with color. Imagine living in a world where everything and everyone are shades of gray: you drink gray water, eat gray food, and hug gray people. Now imagine that all things exist in shades of red: you drink red liquids and eat red foods, and your hair, eyes, and skin are red. Do you think you would feel and interact differently in a monochromatic world than you do in our multichromatic world? Even imagining such a stark reality may have stimulated an emotional reaction that gave you the answer to that question. Probably imagining the gray world elicited dull, flat feelings and the red world gave rise to heightened, faster feelings. You probably would not choose to live in a one-colored world. You are emotionally affected by the multichromatic physical world, and also by the visualized colors of your inner world. Color intention and visualization, as well as seeing color with your physical eyes, transmit distinct physiological, mental, and energetic information throughout your system.

Color is not an easily defined perception, language, or science. It is

211

part of our intuitive language. It heightens perception in daily life and is a core tool in healing and meditation. Color precedes words and antedates civilization, connected as it is to the limbic system of the brain. It is both a subjective experience and an objective feature of the world — both energy and entity. Color is tied to emotions as well as being a physical reality. The intellectual left side of the brain becomes stymied when attempting to describe the experience of color.[1]

From the atmospheric phenomenon of rainbows to the structure of the atom, from the artist's palette to the multihued clothes we wear, color is a key that reflects our physical, emotional, and spiritual world.

COLOR AND SCIENCE

Color is energy made visible.[2]

— John Russell

The source of all color is light. Without light, there is no color. Light is the messenger and color is the message. Leonardo da Vinci observed that color does not exist without light, and was criticized by his peers for such radical thoughts. Robert Boyle, a seventeenth-century English physicist, concluded that colors are diversified light. Isaac Newton demystified the relationship between color and light by passing sunlight through a triangular glass prism; he saw that the rays of white light were bent or refracted, spreading out like a fan. He called the resulting range of colors a spectrum: red, orange, yellow, green, blue, indigo, and violet. He concluded that white light contains all colors, while blackness has none. This analysis of white light was to become one of the most meaningful and famous of all scientific experiments.[3]

We experience color in the world because objects absorb different quantities and frequencies of white light. A green leaf, for instance, contains pigments that absorb certain wavelengths of white light and reflect or transmit others, producing the color of the unabsorbed light: green.

Five discoveries — ranking among the most profound insights in the history of science — were influenced by the study of the color spectrum: the composition of the stars; the relationships among magnetism, electricity, and light; the genesis of quantum mechanics; the structure of the atom; and the expansion of the universe. In 1927, astronomer Edwin Hubble's use of the spectroscope in analyzing the "red planet" established color as a valid, measurable property; from that point onward, color figured into scientific calculations. The spectrum of color thus became a quantifiable constant in scientific measurements. It is interesting to note that Isaac Newton coined the word *spectrum* from a Latin word meaning "apparition." For him, the spectral qualities of color and light occupied a liminal position between this world and another.[4]

In the 1990s, laboratory research using photometers and color filters demonstrated that the human energy field is composed of light/color emissions. Interestingly, the researchers found that the vibrations of the human subtle-energy field did not correspond with biological signals: were as much as a thousand times higher in frequency than the bioelectrical signals of nerve and muscle. To determine the specific color correlations with these signals, professional intuitives observed the auric fields around the bodies of the test subjects while the instruments recorded the signals. The resulting data were subjected to a frequency analysis to determine the frequency spectrum of each color. The resulting comparisons showed that the intuitives' readings correlated with the spectrogram readings at 95 percent accuracy. Further, this research demonstrated that human energy-field colors change rapidly based on will and needs; generally, individuals have a unique, consistent pattern of limited colors (their life force). Only people in peak health and performance had all the colors of the spectrum present in their auras.[5]

COLOR AND CULTURE

Have you had a conversation with someone in which you were both looking at a color but could not agree on the name or shade of that color? This is a historically documented conundrum. The recognition and interpretation of color are determined by many factors — cultural, religious, spiritual, biological, and psychological. The natural development of color recognition is participatory, and the perception of the mind is unconsciously influenced by these factors. For example, ancient Greeks had no word for the color blue, so they described the sea as wine-dark and the sky as bronze. To them, blue was not a color in our sense, but the quality of "darkness." The terms used to describe color were psychological attributes such as "fresh," "dark," "moist," or "alive."[6]

Historical and cultural contexts also influence perception; a Coke bottle dropped from an airplane into a society of Bushmen in South Africa's Kalahari Desert in the movie *The Gods Must Be Crazy* is seen as many things, but never as a container for carbonated beverages. It has been reported that some pre-Columbian Native Americans literally could not see the large sailing vessels of the first European explorers to approach their shores because they had no cultural precedent for such an event or object, and no appropriate words in their vocabulary to describe it. Thus, in their reality, such things simply did not exist.[7] You may be like a European standing next to a Native American, describing a colored aura around a person, to which the Native American replies, "I see nothing." Even the "objective" cognitive act of seeing in the material world requires a synergy of senses.

The human eye can discern the differences among several million variations of hue. *The Pantone Book of Color* displays 1,024 color plates. There are 50,000 different hues (spectral locations), tints, and values of color. In advanced language systems with vast vocabularies, thousands of hues have been given names. But even the most advanced languages contain no more than twelve basic color words.[8] English has eleven basic terms; Russian twelve; the language of New Guinea has two.[9] Many languages have no word for the term *color* itself.[10]

History records color as a silent language used in religion, politics, government, hierarchies, royalty, medicine, war, art, and science. Color wordlessly speaks in allure, authority, beauty, caste, heraldry, marriage, mourning, mysticism, nationalism, nobility, pageantry, patriotism, potency, power, rank, sexuality, and valor.

THE INTUITIVE LANGUAGES OF COLOR AND SOUND

Color is a silent but universal language. Without words and across differing cultures, color can be used for communication among people. Color holds information and transmits messages. Intuitively and instinctively, human memory is stored within a color-coded resonance, like liquid crystal oscillating through the physical and subtle body.

Emotion and memory live in your molecules. They live in the color frequency of your grounding, aura, and chakras. Your energy-colors represent your consciousness. Visualization of color in meditation unlocks stored emotional and psychological information. The color-energy in your body is the container that holds your stories. When you say that your "memory is colored," it may be a literal communication in the practice of Intuition Medicine.

Visualization of color is an intuitive tool to induce healing and orchestrate changes in the arrangement of your energy-information. For example, when you visualize pink life force, you are synchronizing your energy to stimulate and release memories and emotions stored in the pink color frequency. In a healing application, pink life force resonates with love and caring, and therefore injects love-information into your body and energy field. This is like tuning a radio receiver antenna to oscillate at the same frequency as the transmitter in order to receive a specific broadcast of information. This narrows the noise reception to a specific message. In our example, what is being received is the message within the color spectrum of pink. An emotional healing via color meditation can occur instantaneously while you are in a quiet state of mind.

A first-year Intuition Medicine practitioner and veterinarian used color in her meditations to uncover her confusing feelings about love, experienced through her strong dislike of the color pink. She discovered that her aversion to pink was associated with painful childhood memories of incest.

In meditations and in life, the color pink always gave me great trouble, causing a wave of nausea. Working with Intuition Medicine, I discovered that pink brought up both cultural gender issues and memories of my sister's room in childhood, where some not-so-nice things happened for a period of four years. It brought up memories of being "a good little girl in pink." Once I realized the connection and cleansed that energy imprint, I no longer wanted to vomit when I saw or visualized the color pink.

In the intuitive world, it is generally more comprehensible and sensible to agree on a specific language of energy. I find that color works best as a common intuitive language — better than sound, emotions, or electromagnetic signals.

Isaac Newton related the seven colors to the seven notes in an octave, for which he was chided by his colleagues as perpetrating mystical nonsense. But sound was later shown to affect the perception of color. High-pitched tones make colors appear lighter, while low-pitched sounds tend to deepen perceived color. Both the eye and the ear respond to waves of energy.[11] If you are inclined to work with color as frequency, the following table, created by Dr. Valerie Hunt,may be helpful.[12]

COLORS' APPROXIMATE CENTRAL FREQUENCY	
COLOR	APPROXIMATE CENTRAL FREQUENCY IN HERTZ
Low blue	200 Hz
Green	300 Hz
Yellow	400 Hz
Red	500 Hz
Orange	600 Hz
High blue	700 Hz
Violet	800 Hz
Cream	1,000 Hz
White	1,100 Hz and up

If sound, tones, or music stimulate color sensation for you, you can experiment with this table created by Charles Klotsche.[13]

COLOR-SOUND CORRELATIONS		
COLOR	NOTE	SOUND
Red	G	Crickets
Orange	A	Harp
Yellow	A#	Wooden flute
Green	C	Bells/drums
Blue	D	Ocean waves
Indigo	D#	Bees buzzing
Violet	E	Om sound

COLOR, LIGHT, AND ENERGY

Take away the motion of light or color, and we would have no awareness at all of the appearance of matter.[14]

— Roger Lewis

Color is light energy. Energy is stored in light. Matter is frozen light. On the scientific front, light is the cornerstone of quantum mechanics. This new physics postulates that the reality of life is actually light energy that appears solid only because of an illusion created by the mind. Physicist David Bohm summed up this theory in the phrase "All matter is frozen light." With concepts such as these, there is little distinction between the tenets of quantum physics and those of the ancient mystical traditions. The resulting scientific revolution has now given rise to new models of reality in which light has a starring role. Light is powerful and all-encompassing. It constitutes both solid form and life-sustaining energy. Light is fundamental. The artificial lines of separation that we have drawn between physiology and spirituality are blurring; light is their convergence point. There is a growing awareness of the role light plays in maintaining optimal health. Our bodies are biological light receptors. They transform inner light and sunlight into life sustaining energy. However, we have become increasingly removed from both our internal store of light and our external source of light (the sun). Since we have forgotten that light is the core of our being, it is easy to overlook the potential light has to be a formidable ally in the strengthening of life force. Light in the body holds information about health and illness. A lack of sunlight leads to physical malillumination, and a lack of life force leads to spiritual malillumination.[15]

We may ask ourselves: How can light be such an integral part of our reality, scientifically, spiritually, and physically, and not impact our well-being? In fact, light and life are the same energy. When we remember this, we are able to harness the life-sustaining properties of light.[16]

Matter, both dense and subtle, absorbs light and refracts color. The light energy that initiates color sensations has two fundamental dimensions: intensity and wavelength. Intensity determines how bright a light appears. Since light energy is transferred in discrete packets of energy called photons, intensity can be specified in terms of the number of photons that fall on a given area. Newton theorized that rays of light had size. He proposed that light of various colors might be small bodies of various sizes, and that our sensations of color, therefore, were to be understood as our subjective response to the objective reality of the "corpuscular" size of the light's color.[17] Following a Newtonian color-as-size theory, you might experience red as big or green as small.

When you clairvoyantly see color in an aura, it might appear as moving dots of light clustered together. I see these light clusters as uniformly sized corpuscles within each specific color spectrum. When you consistently observe and categorize these packets of light, you can develop a color vocabulary based on this perception of intensity and size. In this way, although you may be unable to see a color in a particular instance, you can recognize the intensity and size of the light — the packets of moving light and the size of the corpuscles — as a particular color.

The wavelength of light is the distance between successive crests in the sine wave. Wavelength determines whether you can see the light with your ocular vision, as well as determining the color sensation it evokes. Light at wavelengths between roughly 400 and 700 nanometers can be absorbed by the photoreceptor cells of the eyes.[18] The rods and cones in your eyeballs absorb this visible light and carry its energy messages to your brain via the optic nerve.

Beyond the 400-to-700-nanometer range of visible light are X-rays and cosmic rays. Interestingly, researchers have documented the human ability to detect cosmic rays with the eye.[19] The degree of functionality of this path of "light news" is determined by a person's genetic makeup (possibly a tetrachromatic gene is responsible), but it can be psychologically altered via cultural influences or physiologically developed via subtle-energy training. Even if you are not born with the genetic sensory system for subtle color perception outside the range of so-called visible light, you can increase your spectral sensitivity to perceive subtle light as color.[20]

Many women in my family have the genetic predisposition to perceive subtle light. However, receptive individuals also need to pay attention to their perceptions when they intuitively register them within, recognize that they perceive more information than most of the people around them, accept the fact that subtle energy is a valid dimension of their experience of reality, and integrate this subtle reality into their lives. If any one of these conditions is not present, the ability may diminish, hamper a person's ability to perceive subtle energy, or create internal chaos.

I accepted my color-seeing as a natural part of sight without question, although I did not realize until my teens that not everyone around me saw subtle light-energy. I feel that my right-brain, introspective, introverted personality maintained my subtle sight at a high degree of functionality. My sister also saw subtle energy in its many forms, but she would not accept the reality of her perceptions. She operated primarily with a left-brain, analytical, extroverted personality. After our mother died, my sister began to see (with her eyes open) our mother's spirit walking through her house. I remember entering my sister's house one day and witnessing her looking disheveled, chain smoking, and pacing frantically. I looked at her energy and saw that our mother's spirit had been visiting her, and that these contacts were disturbing to her. Often people who choose to negate or shut off this perception use prescription and recreational drugs to move out of the realm of subtle reality. The methods used by such naturally sensitive people to keep themselves in dense reality too often become an addictive way of life. Subtle sight can threaten the security of a world built on a culturally agreed-on "sanity." Some decide that it is better to be blind to the preternatural world.

THE PRACTICE OF COLOR HEALING

Colors, like features, follow the changes of the emotions.[21]

— Pablo Picasso

In your Intuition Medicine toolbox, color is a language you can develop based on your own personal and empirical experience.

One Intuition Medicine practitioner found great delight in personalizing her relationship with color:

> *As I practice with colors and the chakra system, I've become aware that colors have "attributes" ascribed to them, but that those qualities or attributes can be mixed and matched. Early on, I used to just stick with rote-learned colors from books for the chakras. Now however, much to my delight, I've discovered that expanding the limits of colors with chakras to include using whatever color feels right for a particular chakra in that moment can be very potent. "Listening" to what color is being called to that chakra is empowering, as I realize that there is an inherent wisdom at work. And then analyzing the color message for its carried information is always humbling and fascinating, as it almost invariably is accurate for the issue that I am working on in my life.*

In the system of Intuition Medicine, the lists of qualities attributed to various colors are collected from thirty years of empirical classroom and clinical data involving thousands of people. The following color list is probably a good base for you to experiment with. In your meditations and healing work, you may find that all applications of the colors elicit the same experiences and results as are found on this list — or you may find your own unique definitions and applications. Your practice of color in healing and meditation is based on your own experience with interpreting each color.

INTUITIVE COLOR ATTRIBUTES	
COLOR	**ATTRIBUTES**
Aqua	Mental and emotional calm
Sky blue	Knowing, intuition, sensitivity, and spirituality
Navy blue	Hypnotic; trancelike
Royal blue	Self-assurance, trust, integrity; indicates physical strength when color is perceived around the body
Cobalt blue	Anesthetic
Teal blue	Soothing panacea
Turquoise blue	Humor, folly, and play
Neutral gray	Doubt, sadness, and depression
Charcoal gray	Somber; earth qualities
Emerald green	Psychic information and intuitive awareness
Forest green	Prosperity and abundance
Apple green	Growth, new information and integration
Red	Passion, courage, physical power, and vitality

COLOR	ATTRIBUTES
Fuchsia	Loving and caring; creative inspiration
Pink	Love, affinity, and humanitarian qualities
Citrus orange	Creative expression and vitality
Burnt orange	Physical health
Peach	Biological healing
Brown	Somber feelings and worry; related to earth
Terra-cotta	Grounding and earth connection
Lavender	Personal spirituality and self-acceptance
Purple	Spiritual seeking and esoteric study
Lemon yellow	Analysis, intellect, and logic
Butter yellow	Abstract intuition
Gold	Embodied harmony, wisdom, and emotional protection
Silver	Personal power
White	Etheric wisdom
Black	Death, fatality, dissolution, and distress; absorptive

COLOR IS IN THE EYE OF THE BEHOLDER

Color is processed differently via the intuitive senses than it is by the brain. Physiological, anatomical, and clinical findings indicate that color is processed in different regions of the brain than those that handle other types of visual information. Surprisingly, the brain cells that transmit color information carry more than one message about the wavelength and spatial distribution of the light and interpret the information by decoding the color through a pooling and comparison of the data.[22] Therefore, it is no wonder that people have difficulty agreeing on a color, shade, or hue. This greatly underscores the need for a consistent, agreed-upon intuitive language of color interpretation based on a common practice and methodology to facilitate communication about color as a language and its use in healing and meditation. Adding to this quandary, most people are able to remember color for only three seconds or three feet, giving "color memory" a very brief recall.[23] Color is truly in the eye, memory, and brain of the beholder.

COLOR IS A MULTISENSORY LANGUAGE

Decoding the energy-message of color may involve a combination of intuitive skills utilized through a multisensory approach — synesthesia. Your pineal gland (associated with clairvoyance) receives and transmits light-energy and is photoreceptive even when your eyes are closed. Humans are photosynthetic (like plants) and absorb light directly through the "solar energy cells" located all over the skin and throughout the body. Meditation with color and light has been used in traditional Chinese medicine to entrain the body's rhythms and to reset the emotional brain for five thousand years.[24] Western medicine recognized light therapy in 1903, when Dr. Niels Finsen was awarded the Nobel Prize in medicine for his work on light and color in healing disease.

Your skin is your largest sense organ, and because it is also photoreceptive, you can think of it as dermal optics — you can see color via any area of your skin! It is possible to learn how to perceive the color of pieces of paper or other objects through sensations in your hands. Your hands and the skill of psychometry are the most commonly utilized intuitive synergy of touch and seeing receptors, but any area of your skin may also be as photoreceptive. Interestingly, the skin emits thirty photons per square centimeter per second.[25] There is also evidence that infrared radiation and microwaves are emitted from the body.[26] This would provide enough light for a photosensitive person to see the human energy field in the dark. Using your hands to detect energy — psychometry — increases your clairvoyance. Brain waves are conducted from the fingers to the brain via the perineural and circulatory systems. This data validates what I have observed for years — that utilizing psychometry in energy work stimulates and develops clairvoyance.

Many people can hear color — about one woman in twenty and fewer men. That is to say, sounds produce mental sensations of color for them.[27] Pay attention; color may be singing to you! Maybe that is what Walt Whitman was referring to when he wrote, "I sing the body electric."[28]

In your practice, begin to develop intuitive color perception by meditating with your eyes closed; this disconnects the information pathway from the optic nerve to the brain.[29] Eventually, you will be able to distinguish the brain-decoded message of color from the intuitive perception of color. I suggest that you use a blend of intuitive skills to perceive color via synesthesia: psychometry with clairvoyance, clairsentience with knowing, and so forth. Color perception is in the eyes, hands, ears, and skin of the beholder. When you are in a store looking at rows of bottles of vitamin C and cannot decide which brand will work best for you, try this fun experiment. Place your hands about 3 inches in front of the row of bottles and move your hands slowly in front of them. The psychometric detection in your hands will register an energy signal reporting which vitamin C is in affinity with you. Similarly, the subtle-energy (light) emissions of food tell us how much life force it contains.

A common language for describing color requires more than functional physical organs. Without the inner light of a formative visual imagination, we are all blind. *New Scientist* magazine reports that new ways of probing the brain are transforming the established view of sensory perception, yielding the current consensus that we have at least twenty-one senses; and that the boundaries between them are blurred.[30] The idea that our sensations are determined by the sensory organ that picks up the information is being challenged.

PRACTICAL COLOR HEALING IN DAILY LIFE

How much are you influenced by color in your life? I recall two vivid experiences. The first was seeing the awe-inspiring spectacle of a triple rainbow in the American desert. The second was clairvoyantly seeing a uniquely colored aura. In this second case, I was on a boat in the Caribbean Islands, taking bell-diving lessons. I was mesmerized by the instructor's highly unusual green aura — a green that I had never seen. Actually, his entire energy system was this unique green, with no trace of any other color. When it was my turn to jump off the boat with him and submerge, I was stunned to see that everything underwater was that same unique algae-green color! This lifelong diver had immersed himself so completely in his aquatic reality that he had thoroughly matched his aura to the color frequency of this specific algae-green underwater world.

Your daily moods are influenced by color in your environment, the colors of food, nature, and all the other objects around you. All these colors have a potentially monumental influence on your well-being. You can discriminatingly manage their influence by observing and applying your intuitive color awareness. Eat a rainbow diet — a daily menu of many differently colored foods, as prescribed by Dr. Gabriel Cousins in his book *Spiritual Nutrition and the Rainbow Diet.*[31] Surround yourself with colors you love. Try on different colors in your aura and clothing as you walk through life, and observe their effect on you. Consciously use color throughout your daily activities to create the most comfortable environment in which to live.

Here are some daily situations and color solutions from Intuition Medicine practitioners:

Occasionally I am with an individual or a group and feel disagreeable pressures. In this situation, I first try to determine what color or colors that group or individual is emanating. Then I try to energetically match it or use a complementary hue.

A pony I was working with was extremely nervous and would not calm down. So I decided I would touch-heal the pony with an earthy brown color so that he would ground better and feel more comfortable about the situation. Sure enough, after no more than five minutes, the pony became calm and gave amazingly gentle rides to children at a party.

In my artwork, I meditate on which color best represents the emotional energy of the art piece I am working on, and then I work with that color.

When I enter a room that feels uncomfortable, I visualize a comforting color and fill the room with that color. The mood usually changes immediately.

I visualize my essence colors in my aura in order to flow more easily with a group that I am not in energetic harmony with. This gives me confidence to be myself.

When I am feeling sad or out of sorts and want to change my mood to a more uplifting level, I intend that my personal healing colors surround and fill me.

During my five-minute walk to work, I fill myself up with a color. It is eye-opening to see the powerful effect on me and the people I meet during the walk. This is a great way for me to set my mood for the day!

I was standing in front of my acrobatics equipment at the circus school where I teach, with no inspiration or energy to do anything. I started meditating with red and orange — fire colors — and within a couple of minutes, I was inspired to create a new aerial acrobatics routine.

I often surround myself with gold energy as a personal protection against other energies and to mirror healing to those around me.

I get nervous when I have to speak in front of a group. I had to address a large group at a recent board meeting. These people were incredibly successful financially and were educated at prestigious institutions. I was feeling a little intimidated, or at least experiencing some performance anxiety. Half an hour before my presentation, I went into the storage room in my office. I began to meditate, ground, and heighten my life-force energy with brilliant colors; then I created a rainbow of energy around my aura. Feeling vibrant and relaxed, I entered the conference room and delivered my presentation with confidence and without butterflies in my stomach or a crackly voice. The response was extremely favorable, with several members seriously considering an addition to my budget.

I visualize a blue egg with pink inside it around me. I affirm that only har-
monious, positive energies reach me and that all negative energy is repelled.
I am astounded by the power and simplicity of using color to establish an
effective boundary.

One morning, I encountered a situation that made me very angry. I was
not sure what color my aura was, but I bet it was red because I feel the same
fiery feeling when I meditate with red. I tried to change my aura to pink,
but it was too drastic a change. Instead, I tried hot pink, which still felt pas-
sionate but took the edge off. Then I proceeded to rectify the situation that
had angered me. I could deal with people in a direct yet respectful way and
communicate my grievances without blaming anyone. I was able to clear
up the problem in this way.

In the 1970s, when I was a medical intuitive at the Academy of Eastern Medicine, we created a color healing system for the clinic patients
using chromotherapy and color meditation. The practice of chromotherapy involves using colored gel slides inserted over a lamp. The patient
would lie down on a table and the colored light would bathe the area of
the body being treated. The choice of color and length of the color bath
were determined by the clinic medical doctor, a neurologist who was also
trained in chromotherapy and ayurvedic medicine. I would follow this
treatment with a guided color visualization meditation, which would be
tape-recorded and given to the patient as daily meditation/medication.
This dual procedure of color meditation and chromotherapy proved to be
an efficacious treatment for a variety of problems: nervous system disor-
ders, high blood pressure, pain management, and skin conditions.[32]
It is now common hospital practice to give jaundiced babies blue-
light baths rather than blood transfusions. In general, it has been found
that blue light lessens newborn crying and overactivity. However, the blue
light irritates nurses working in these wards, and many hospitals add gold
lamps to impart a soothing quality.[33] If you have prayed in a church with
colored stained-glass windows while the light streamed through and
bathed you in resplendent colors, you were partaking in an ancient
chromo-healing ritual.

CONTEMPLATIVE COLOR MEDITATION

When the body is in a normal condition, it filters out from the white light or sunlight whatever color vibration it needs. However, if a person is not in normal health, the necessary color must be supplied.[34]

— C. G. Sander

In meditation practice (see the next chapter), color resonates with a rhythmic pulsation that entrains your energy to respond to the information-laden hue. The concept and practice of entrainment are important to understand in order to receive the intended healing outcome. *Entrainment* is a term used in physics to describe a situation in which two similar frequencies become coupled with each other until they both vibrate at the same frequency. For example, two pendulum clocks set next to each other eventually synchronize their swings, and women living together find that their menstrual periods eventually synchronize to the same time of the month. In meditation, our energy can be entrained when our brain waves are in a free-run or silent period — that is, when they are uncoupled from the entrained brain frequency and susceptible to external influence. In meditation, the "influence" is the intentional visualization of color. This free-run or quiet state of mind, or still-point period, occurs intermittently and lasts from five to twenty-five seconds.[35] Therefore, a full minute or more of focused meditation, in repeated sessions, is necessary for any sustained healing outcome to occur. This is the transformative occurrence that many refer to as the "healing state of mind."

Meditation slows our brain waves, creating greater coherence among all the frequency oscillations in our systems. This releases us from physical and mental perceptions, producing expanded perception during all the still points. In this state of expanded subjective time, we can better absorb, collect, and manifest information. That is why being in a quiet, meditative state of mind is so powerful and effective.[36]

LIVING IN COLOR

I sensed a scream passing through nature. I painted... the clouds as actual blood. The colour shrieked.[37]

— Edvard Munch, on his painting *The Scream*

Do you hear color? Does it shriek, laugh, and cry? Do you feel color as happy, sad, or calm? Can you taste color as a quality? Does color affect you spiritually, psychologically, and physically?

Color in meditation is a tool for self-healing, releasing blocks, restoring vitality, tapping into information, and providing emotional protection. Color can alter moods and subtly communicate emotions. All people radiate color around themselves and throughout their physical bodies. Everyone has "essence colors" in their energy field that display their core personalities. Most of your essence colors remain the same throughout your life, while your mood colors shift according to your circumstances. Have you been "red with anger" or "in the pink" — or maybe "green with envy" or enveloped by a "gray cloud"? Many people feel in color and use color to describe their emotions. You have probably felt unspoken joy or sadness emanating from other people; the human energy field emits moods, carried on a color-light-information frequency like an emotive telegraph message.

The effect of color in meditation falls into one or more of the following categories:

- Physical and material: colors that affect the body and the material world

- Vital and power-giving: colors that impart strength and the ability to perform or act effectively

- Mental and psychological: colors that open and stimulate the mind and psyche

- Harmonizing and unifying: colors that create a mood of calm or well-being

- Specific healing: colors that have a defined use

- Inspiration and intuition: colors that open and access psychic and creative senses

- Spiritual and of a higher consciousness: colors that expand one's perceptions of God/Goddess or the Divine

PERSPECTIVES ON COLOR

I see colors in the aura as a reflection of the soul and the spirit, the mind and the body.[38]

— Edgar Cayce

Your perspective on color and your experiences with it are valuable teaching tools. Create a daily and weekly chart of the colors you meditate with — those you use as healing tools — and the color moods you experience during the day. You can chart colors before and after meditation, after a day of work, after lovemaking, when feeling stress, on a good day, and so forth. Experiment with adjusting your color frequently during the day, then compare your moods and experiences. You will learn a tremendous amount about how you are affected and how your conscious manipulation of color can change your reality.

Reflections and Journaling

From your daily-life experiences as well as your meditations, give each of your colors a personal word to describe its mood or quality. Here are some frequently used color-description words: alien, calming, cleansing, cold, dirty, dull, dynamic, earthy, expansive, familiar, fast, feminine, fertile, flat, fuzzy, happy, hard, harmonious, harsh, hot, jagged, loud, masculine, neutral, nurturing, passionate, peaceful, powerful, quiet, regal, restful, robust, rough, sacred, sensual, serious, slow, smooth, soft, spiritual, sterile, strong, subtle, sunny, tranquil, vital, weak.

Journaling

Because there are no absolutes in the study of the human energy field, you will find that some entries in the following lists overlap with or are the same as entries on other chapter lists. When cross-referencing your personal journal lists, you may find repetitive or similar entries; this indicates a theme or a lesson for you to pay attention to in the management of your energy. Use personal experience and discernment in your assessment of all the entries.

HOW IT FEELS WHEN YOUR ENERGY-COLORS ARE...	
IN HARMONY	**OUT OF HARMONY**
The color immediately appears during meditation or with intention	The color is dark, black, or mixed with a murky color
The color resonates with your body	The color appears fragmented or not fully formed
It is effortless to see, experience, and embrace the color	You have difficulty integrating the color
You feel empowered and uplifted by the color's healing properties	There is a distortion of the frequency
You experience a natural attraction to and resonance with the color	You feel general discomfort when attempting to hold the color's vibration
The color cleanses your energy or brings in the desired application effectively	The color brings up uncomfortable feelings or memories
The color feels good in your body; it looks bright and positive	The color feels distasteful or incongruent
You sense an internal validation	Application of the color to an area creates disharmony
When filling up your chakras or other systems with the color, you feel calm	There is a feeling of effort with the application
All your body energies feel like they are vibrating at a comfortable and joyous rate	The color is dull or lacks luster
	The color feels draining or life-taking; there is a basic discordant feeling
The color is easily absorbed into your body and/or energy systems	When filling up chakras, the color creates dissonant feelings
The color looks or feels in synchrony with your systems	The color creates agitation
	The color ungrounds a system
	The color feels oppressive or suppressive
	The color dissipates or disappears in application

Reflections

Take a moment to think about the following self-reflective questions. Trust the first insights that come to you as your intuitive answers.

- Think about times in your life when you have noticed indications of color in your energy field; what were you doing then?

- Think about times in your life when you have noticed indications of color in other people's energy fields; what activity were you engaged in when you intuited this color information?

Using your color perceptions as an intuitive language of information, you can become more aware of subtle communications and messages when you interact with others. Next time you notice any perception of energy-color, stop and interpret the meaning of the color message in relation to the immediate interaction, thoughts, or situation. Your color perceptions are a subtle language that validates your active involvement in intuitive communication. Learn to notice and act on these color messages and perceptions, and you will be using a universal human language.

ARE YOU AWARE OF YOUR ENERGY-COLOR HEALTH NEEDS?

The purest and most thoughtful minds are those which love color the most.[39]

— John Ruskin

Color as energy is information. Diagnostic health information is provided by the intensity of color in a person's energy field: bright colors indicate mental harmony, a healthy body and mind, and happy moods; pale, cloudy, or murky colors indicate dissonant emotions, a tired and unhealthy body, or sad moods. When you visualize bright colors in your meditations, you are working toward raising the health vibration of your energy. You then naturally raise the health vibration of your body, mind, and spirit. The body stores color vibration in the way that electrical potential is stored in a battery — waiting to be drawn on when needed to maintain an optimum level of life-force energy.

The lists following contain information about how the qualities of colors affect healing and the use of specific colors in particular healing applications. The information in these lists is compiled from thirty years of empirical classroom and clinical data, involving thousands of people. It also has been cross-referenced with information about other subtle-energy systems. As color can be a personal, subjective energy experience, you might agree or disagree with these entries.

TRANSLATION OF COLOR QUALITIES FOR HEALING	
COLORS ENHANCE A STATE OF HEALTH WHEN THEY ARE...	COLORS DEPLETE A STATE OF HEALTH WHEN THEY ARE...
High amperage	Low amperage
Full of light	Dark, without light
Translucent	Opaque
Clear	Murky
Bright	Dissipated
Pure	Static
Vital	Flat
Coherent	Chaotic
Held with an intention for greater good	Held with an intention to do harm
COLORS ENHANCE A STATE OF HEALTH WHEN THEY ORIGINATE FROM...	COLORS DEPLETE A STATE OF HEALTH WHEN THEY ORIGINATE FROM...
Your essence energy	Electrical equipment
God/Goddess energy	Your or another's negative thoughts
Divine guidance	Other people's energy (near or far)
Light, unchanged by emotion or thought	Light in a state of entropy

COLORS WITH APPLICATIONS FOR HEALING AND MEDITATION	
COLOR	**APPLICATION**
Cobalt blue	Anesthetizes
Gold and copper	Cleanses unhealthy memories and emotions
Platinum	Induces out-of-body experiences
Pearlescent violet	Connects to universal abundance
Golden white (pearl)	Connects to universal consciousness
Rose-gold	Buddha/Christ healing energy
Black pearl	Induces access to mystical realms
Clear or crystalline	Amplifies energy
Ice/glacier blue	Stops flow of kundalini energy
Metallic color(s)	Brings clarity to kundalini energy
Rainbow obsidian	Induces astral/dream travel

Think about the preceding lists and reflect on these questions:

- How does the "enhance and deplete" information compare to your experience of energy and color, both in meditation and as it surrounds you in your home, life, work, and so forth?

- Are you more attracted to "enhance" or "deplete" colors?

- Do you use the "enhance" or "deplete" colors in your healing meditations, and do you resonate in the "enhance" or "deplete" color range?

- What is your experience with the applications in the "Healing and Meditations" lists? Do you agree or disagree with the listed usages?

Take a moment to think about these questions and write your responses in your journal. As you become more aware of how color affects you, you will be able to immediately change your energy-colors to alter your mood and state of mind. This will help you come into an awareness of the profound effect that color has on your physical, psychological, and spiritual health.

I hope that this chapter on color has given you a new way to look at human communication and stimulated a practical perspective on living life in a body of health.

When you feel ready to put what you have learned from this chapter into a language of intuition, go to the next chapter, "The Color Meditation and Healing Practice," and practice using color as a language and a healing tool.

Chapter 15

THE COLOR MEDITATION
AND HEALING PRACTICE

The rainbow mirrors human aims and action.

Think, and more clearly wilt thou grasp it, seeing

Life is but light in many-hued reflection.

— Johann Wolfgang von Goethe

The focus of the color practice is to give you simple, powerful tools that guide you to know, feel, and perceive energy-color; to develop your ability to diagnose your health via energy-color; and to use color as a healing tool. Color as intuitive language is essential to the practice of Intuition Medicine and further strengthens your ability to use intuition as a natural human sense. When you practice color perception as intuitive sight, you strengthen your clairvoyant and diagnostic skills.

Contemplative Meditations

There are two color meditations in this chapter. The rainbow meditation is designed to guide you in perceiving and feeling the energy of color as mood and sensation — the emotional-intuitive language of your body. This is a good meditation to practice in order to strengthen and establish color as a tool for managing and shifting your moods, as well as to recover your stored memories. The second meditation combines color with grounding, the meditation sanctuary, life-force and earth energy, the aura, and the chakras in a complete energy-systems meditation.

You may choose to do the two meditations one after the other or to do one at a time. Take time to reflect on your experiences with each color meditation. After each of the meditations, follow the post-meditation questions as a guide for further discovery; write notes on your personal reflections in your journal.

Rainbow Meditation

Choose a list of colors to work with during each rainbow meditation. You might use the colors from the "Intuitive Color Attributes" chart on pages 223–224 or create a personal list of your favorite colors. Also, you can gather swatches of fabric, gems and minerals, or colored paint chips from a paint or art-supply store to hold in your hands. If you practice with a colored object in your hands while you visualize that same color, you will develop psychometry and clairvoyance to operate in synesthesia perception.

- Begin by grounding yourself and resting your attention in your meditation sanctuary.

- Visualize each color as a waterfall of light above you, flowing into your head, filling your body, and radiating around you, filling your aura with a corona of light. Hold the feelings for a quiet moment. Then, in intuitive inquiry, focus on the following:

  - Perceive any subtle change of mood or feelings; describe it with a word.

  - Is the color's vibration fast or slow, heavy or light, hot or cold, dense or shallow?

  - Notice whether the color feels familiar.

  - If the color is familiar, does it evoke memories of people, places, activities, or symbols?

  - Do you feel the color in your body? If so, locate the specific area(s) where you feel it.

- Do you like or dislike the color sensation or experience?

- Are you comfortable or uncomfortable with the color?

- Follow these steps with each color on your list.

- Compare each successive color with the one before it by sensing whether the color is faster/slower, heavier/lighter, hotter/cooler, or deeper/shallower. This will give you personal relational information about the action of each color on your body and subtle-energy field.

Grounding, Meditation Sanctuary, Life-Force and Earth Energy, Aura, Chakra, and Color Meditation

This is a long meditation. Prepare yourself by finding a quiet place and a comfortable seat.

- Close your eyes and begin to breathe slowly, inhaling through your nose and exhaling through your mouth. Breathe with the intention of slowing down and relaxing. Focus on listening to the sound of your breath. Do this for about a minute, then let your breathing return to a natural rhythm.

- Be present in your meditation sanctuary. Greet yourself and listen to your inner voice.

- With your attention in your meditation sanctuary, intuitively inquire, "What color(s) is healing for my grounding?"

- You may receive answers via knowing, psychometry, clairvoyance, clairaudience, telepathy, clairsentience, or a combination of your intuitive abilities. Trust your first insight, and visualize or hold the intention of that color(s) filling your energy field.

- Continue the intuitive inquiry for each of your energy systems: "What color(s) is healing for my ____?" Focus this inquiry on your grounding, life-force and earth energy, aura and chakras. You may also include your physical body systems in this color meditation.

- Trust your first insight and visualize or hold the intention of that color(s) filling each system. Affirm that the highest healing energy information resonates within each system.

- For each energy system, affirm a healing intention and hold the color-meditation setting for a quiet moment.

- After color-healing all the energy systems, bring energetic closure to your systems by clasping your hands together or wrapping your arms around your body in a hug.

- Sit in quiet repose.

Observational Practices: Post-Meditation Questions

Directly after a meditation is a good time to write any immediate feelings, thoughts, or insights in your journal. The eight following questions will help you integrate color as an intuitive tool into your healing and meditation practice.

1. How did each of the colors make you feel?

2. Did any of the colors especially attract you?

3. Did any of the colors make you feel uncomfortable?

4. Did you have difficulty visualizing any of the colors?

5. Choose two of the colors from the meditation and consider how you might use them in your daily practice and your daily life.

6. Could you sense your essence colors? If so, what were they?

7. Which colors were transitional mood colors? Which moods did they correspond to?

8. Was specific information associated with any colors? Did you see symbols or words or get a knowing sense of information with any colors?

Daily-Living Tips

- Notice the colors you are drawn to throughout the day. Be aware of the emotional and physical effects of specific external colors.

- Intuit the presence of colors during specific moods, and change them as you choose.

- Intuit the colors that can shift you out of less desirable moods, and proactively integrate them into your daily life.

- As you interact with others during your day, notice the colors they are emitting and whether they affect you.

- Change your color(s) in your aura and in the clothes you wear to increase social harmony and personal well-being.

Experiments: Try This!

Hands are a rich source of energy-information, as well as sensitive detection tools for diagnosis and healing. This therapeutic-touch exercise develops psychometry and clairvoyance.

- Begin by grounding yourself and resting your attention in your meditation sanctuary.

- Visualize a color as a waterfall of light above you, flowing into your head, filling up your body, and radiating around you, filling your aura with a corona of light. Hold the feelings for a quiet moment.

- Place the palms of your hands facing each other, without touching, about six inches apart.

- Create a ball of energy between your hands and fill it with that specific color-energy. Move your hands farther apart and closer together, enlarging and shrinking the ball of energy.

- As you hold the ball of color between your hands, find words to describe or give a quality to the feeling of the color.

- Repeat the steps with a rainbow of colors.

- For a therapeutic-touch color treatment, place your hand(s) on a specific area and visualize the color running through your hands into the area until you feel saturation (via surplus energy pushing back at your hand or overheating of the area) or you know that the energy transmission is complete. Hold an intention for the specific color application. For example, if you are treating pain in your shoulder, meditate with cobalt blue and then place your hand(s) on your shoulder as you affirm that the pain is releasing.

And Try This!

- For a mood-altering experience, experiment with color by immersing yourself in a bath of colored water and adding the same color of bathroom lighting. You might add persimmon juice to the water for red or spinach juice for green, or float pink rose petals or yellow daisies in the water. Use the same color of lightbulb in the bathroom. This is a subtle and fun experience!

Affirmations: Repeat Often

- I listen to and honor my quiet, inner knowing.

- I am in harmony and collaboration with the universe.

- I create my personal reality.

- I see the beauty of life in the colors of the world.

- Each day, I welcome the color energy that is in highest harmony with my health and well-being.

Trust

Practice discernment as it brings forth an authentic life. Listen deeply to your inner wisdom and to the authentic voices of others. You have the capacity for more life, love, and wisdom.

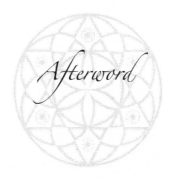

Afterword

Wellness is available for those who go beyond logic to common sense.

— C. Norman Shealy and Caroline Myss

$\mathcal{B}$*ody of Health* is meant to be placed in your library alongside other health reference volumes. Use this book as a map for emotional, physical, and spiritual healing practices; to find new insight on energetic causes of dis-ease; to create a shift in your perspective on relationships; and to be reminded that health is grounded in following your practical intuition. Your body is filled with health-medicine, and intuition is the interpretive language of your inner pharmacopoeia of well-being. The information in this book articulates a healthy-living, personal, everyday practice.

You are your best inner physician, and this book is your *materia medica* — book of health. I suggest you read *Body of Health* several times with particular goals:

• First read the book to find new information about health, energy, and self-care.

- Get serious about studying sections that you feel will support you in personal healing and assist you in maintaining a sense of well-being.

- Choose practice chapters that appeal to you, and work with the contemplative instructions to develop a meditation practice.

- Record a meditation tape from a practice chapter by reading the step-by-step instructions into a tape recorder. Or purchase my voice-guided audio set through my website at www.intuition medicine.org.

- Make a list of the affirmations from the practice chapters and post the lists at home, at work, or wherever you spend time. Read them often as part of your daily practice of positive thinking.

- Carry an Intuition Medicine journal with you and write down immediate intuitive insights you have during the day. Later, read the appendixes chakra lists and find descriptions that match your insights. This creates a living language of intuition directly relevant to your life experiences.

- Carry copies of the Aura and Chakra Illustration for Diagnosis and Journaling on page 203 and colored pencils, pens, or crayons with you to work, on vacations, when visiting friends, and so forth. Pull them out at various times and quickly draw in the energy, information, colors, symbols, and other elements that you intuit in your body, chakras, aura and grounding. Later, use the information lists in this book to translate and interpret the meanings of your drawing.

- Read *Body of Health* once a year as a reminder to renew your healthy-living perspective.

The wisdom tools in this book are integral to the health of your relationships. Give friends a copy and start a dialogue about your understanding of the material and how you operate with your intuitive sense; this creates human engagement, bringing more discernment and further knowledge to the journey of whole human living.

Learning within a group can be a powerful experience. Consider bringing a few like-minded people together to focus on a chapter of the book each week. Work with the information and exercises together in the form of discussions or hands-on practice. You might also find a school or teacher who can instruct you in becoming familiar with the connection between wellness and intuition; this is a powerful prescription for health. If you live in California's San Francisco Bay Area, join our Academy of Intuition Medicine program; if you live outside Northern California, you can enroll in our distance education program. Knowledge acquisition, whether alone or with a group, is a wisdom-laden excursion.

Life is an exploratory journey of health, balance, and energy; a good map helps you find your way with ease and grace. Thank you for reading my map!

With Good Thoughts,
Francesca
Marin County, 2005

Appendix 1

INTUITION MEDICINE HEALTH ISSUES REFERENCE CHART

A Physician must be a Philosopher; that is to say, he must dare to use his own reason and not cling to antiquated opinions and book-authorities. He must above all be in possession of that faculty which is called Intuition, and which cannot be acquired by blindly following the footsteps of another; he must be able to see his own way. The Physician who wants to know man must look upon him as a whole and not as a patched-up piece of work. If he finds a part of the human body diseased, he must look for the causes that produce the disease, and not merely treat the external effects. Philosophy — the true perception and understanding of cause and effect — is the mother of the Physician, and explains the origin of all his diseases.

— Paracelsus

HOW TO USE THE CHART

*I*ntuition Medicine gives you the ability to maintain a healthy body and state of mind by accessing your inner physician. The practitioners of this system of healing have observed that with regular, consistent practice, the health of the immune system is strengthened, many minor ailments disappear, and cyclical illness does not occur or is greatly diminished. When an illness originates at the energy level, you can choose to work with your inner pharmacopoeia of medicine and meditate to heal the issue. Some of the most common energy-based health problems can be remedied easily with practice: pain located around chakras, headaches, sadness, anxiety, eyestrain, stomachache, bloating, constipation, and irregular menses.

The educational objectives of this practice include:

- acquiring wisdom, utilizing the language of intuition

- gathering energy-information through meditation

- comprehending the meaning of your energy-information

- analyzing the application of energy as a healing tool

- creating a personal healing and meditation practice that is a synthesis of your intuitive wisdom gathering

Intuition Medicine gives you a contemplative and daily-awareness life practice for health and harmony of body, mind, and spirit. One benefit of this practice is developing the ability to recognize how your personal state of energy and health feel, in contrast to a diminished state of well-being. As you develop your body of health, you craft a tool to maintain a positive-energy protection field around your sensitive body. You achieve a heightened sense of intuition. Personal spiritual growth occurs, and you realize the oneness of your body, mind, and spirit. With regular practice, you feel happy without being perfect. Centered in the midst of chaos, you are emotionally grounded and you live in your body. You walk through your life with ease and grace, enjoying the present moment.

The "Health Issues Reference Chart" is a documentary collection of data, not a set of medical prescriptions. The health issues listed represent the conditions that I have studied in my practice of energy medicine and Intuition Medicine, involving thousands of clients and students over the past thirty years. The healing advice includes the most common applications that have yielded positive results for each of the health issues listed. In order to more clearly follow the suggestions as they have been used in practice, specific directions are indicated for each health issue.

In the color column of the chart, the indicated color(s) is recommended for visualizing your life-force energy and applying it throughout your energy and physical anatomy systems. In the grounding, life-force, and earth-energy columns, "Need more" indicates a lack of the specific energy; you need to visualize more of that particular energy in your practice. In the aura column, "Need to strengthen" indicates a weak aura condition; the vital force is lacking around the body, and the auric energy force needs to be strengthened throughout the entire cocoon of energy surrounding the body. In the meditation sanctuary column, "Be there" means just that! If you are not located in your meditation sanctuary, you need to affirm or visualize your primary attention as more fully present in that location.

For each specific chakra indicated in relation to a given health issue, visualize the suggested color(s) resonating in the suggested chakra(s). If a single color is indicated, that is the primary healing color vibration. If two colors are listed with a plus sign (+), use both, either separately or woven together; two colors with a dash (-) between them means you are advised to weave the two colors together. For a few health issues, the chart directs you to use one specific color, then follow it with a second, separate color, rather than to weave the two together. "Rainbow" means to visualize as many colors as possible — a plethora of rich color vibrations.

You are an eternal student of life. I recommended that you use the information offered here as a starting place for your own self-healing practice. Listen to your intuition and adjust the recommendations as you incorporate this information into your health practice. Trust your intuition and follow through on it as you engage your inner physician.

The "Health Issues Reference Chart" is not a source of absolute diagnostic advice, nor is it to be used in lieu of a doctor's advice. Intuition Medicine is an integrative practice; in order for you to receive optimum benefit, you need to combine this practice with diagnosis and prescriptive advice from qualified physicians. The body has physical lessons to learn, and the spirit has lessons of the soul to learn — both of equal value. This chart and the material in this book are not intended as medical advice. If you have a medical condition or issue, consult a qualified physician.

INTUITION MEDICINE HEALTH ISSUES REFERENCE CHART

HEALTH ISSUES	CHAKRA	COLOR	GROUNDING	AURA
Abdominal pain	3rd	Cobalt blue		Need to strengthen
Alcoholism; drug abuse	1st and 7th	Purple or blue	Need more	
Angina; arteriosclerosis	4th	Red		
Anorexia; bulimia	3rd	Yellow		
Anxiety, stress	1st and 3rd	Earth colors		Need to strengthen
Arthritis	2nd and 5th	Fuchsia + orange		
Asthma	1st and 4th	Pink		Need to strengthen
Bladder issues	2nd	Blue, then orange		
Bone and skeletal issues	1st	Cobalt blue, then burnt orange		
Bronchitis	5th	Orange		
Colds	Heal all	Rainbow		Need to strengthen
Colitis	1st	Orange		Need to strengthen
Coma	1st and 7th	Lavender-pearl	Need more	
Constipation; diarrhea	1st and 2nd	Yellow		
Depression	1st, 4th, and 7th	Pink	Need more	Need to strengthen
Ear Issues	5th and telepathic	Golden-white		Need to strengthen

MEDITATION SANCTUARY	LIFE-FORCE ENERGY	EARTH ENERGY	HAND CHAKRAS	FEET CHAKRAS	TELEPATHIC CHAKRAS
		Need more			
e there					
	Need more	Need more			
			100%		
			50–100%		
		Need more			
	Need more				
	Need more	Need more			
	Need more	Need more			
		Need more			
e there	Need more	Need more			
	Need more				10–20%

INTUITION MEDICINE HEALTH ISSUES REFERENCE CHART

HEALTH ISSUES	CHAKRA	COLOR	GROUNDING	AURA
Eczema	1st and 4th	Blue + pink		Need to strengthen
Edema	2nd	Sky blue		
Eye issues	7th or telepathic	Earth colors	Need more	
Headaches	6th, 7th, or telepathic	Cobalt blue	Need more	
High blood pressure	1st and 4th	Sky blue	Need more	Need to strengthen
Insomnia	1st, 3rd, and 7th 20%	Gold		
Kidney issues	1st and 3rd	Purple	Need more	
Liver issues	1st and 2nd	Yellow		
Menopause	1st, 2nd, and 7th	Peach	Need more	
Mental confusion	7th 10–20%	Red	Need more	
Reproductive system: female	1st, 2nd, and 7th	Orange	Need more	
Reproductive system: male	1st, 2nd, and 3rd	Red	Need more	
Sciatica	1st and feet chakras	Sky blue, then cobalt blue	Need more	
Stomach issues	3rd	Green		Need to strengthen
Thyroid issues	5th	Burnt orange	Need more	
Ulcers	1st and 3rd	Pink, then cobalt blue		
Vertigo	7th 10–20%	Gold	Need more	

MEDITATION SANCTUARY	LIFE-FORCE ENERGY	EARTH ENERGY	HAND CHAKRAS	FEET CHAKRAS	TELEPATHIC CHAKRAS
e there					10–20%
	Need more				
e there		Need more			10%
e there					10–20%
	Need more				
	Need more	Need more			
e there	Need more	Need more			
e there		Need more		100%	
	Need more	Need more			
	Need more	Need more			
				100%	
e there	Need more	Need more			
				100%	

Appendix 2
CHAKRA SYSTEM REFERENCE CHARTS

$\mathcal{T}$he following charts are compiled from two hundred questionnaires completed by Intuition Medicine practitioners, with an age range of twenty to seventy years old (median age: thirty-six), who regularly practiced this methodology for two to ten years. The first chart lists answers to the question "During what activities/occasions do you dial down/ open up this chakra?" The second chart lists answers to the question "How do you know when your chakras are in harmony/out of harmony?" These charts are added to the chakra material contained in the chapters in order to give you more comprehensive information about how to work with chakras in daily awareness practice.

WHEN TO DIAL DOWN OR OPEN UP YOUR CHAKRAS		
CHAKRA	DURING WHICH ACTIVITIES DO YOU DIAL DOWN THIS CHAKRA?	DURING WHICH ACTIVITIES DO YOU OPEN UP THIS CHAKRA?
1st	Cleansing, clearing, or grounding the chakra Feeling vulnerable, threatened, fearful, anxious, unsafe, or panicking In survival mode Feeling off balance In new places In a poverty mindset Involved with transportation (cars, airplanes) Experiencing energy invasion or energy leaks Someone is grounding through you Setting up or giving a consultation/meditation/healing Dealing with parents, children, or family situations Working with clients In crowds Getting ready for bed Wanting to allow the greater meditative energies of upper chakras to concentrate their effect Around strongly single-minded people Needing protection against negativity Experiencing menses or PMS Feeling unwell Not being in present time Feeling sleepy but needing to stay alert Under stress	Wanting to connect with the earth or to ground Wanting to restore health Resolving financial matters Searching for new career choices Wanting to feel secure and safe Exercising or doing dangerous activity Involved in emergency situations Cleansing or clearing the chakra or clearing emotional energy

	WHEN TO DIAL DOWN OR OPEN UP YOUR CHAKRAS	
CHAKRA	DURING WHICH ACTIVITIES DO YOU DIAL DOWN THIS CHAKRA?	DURING WHICH ACTIVITIES DO YOU OPEN UP THIS CHAKRA?
2nd	Needing to boost emotional neutrality; taking on or feeling someone else's emotions (empathy or sympathy); emotionally out of balance; needing emotional control or protection; being around emotional people or situations; feeling emotionally sick; being around untrustworthy people Feeling overly clairsentient Experiencing energy invasion or energy leaks Feeling sympathetic pains of clients stuck in your body In teaching/learning situations or neutral situations Being in a hurry Setting up or during a consultation/meditation/healing Meeting new people or being in large groups In work meetings Around children or family Someone is attempting to energy-merge Needing to diminish inappropriate attention from someone Wanting to diminish unwanted sexual attraction; preventing others from leeching sexual energy In a toxic environment	Needing to cleanse or clear the chakra or clear emotional energy Involved in a consultation/meditation/healing Wanting to heal sexual organs Connecting into and communicating with the body Focusing on and feeling sensual energy; intimacy or sexual activity with a trusted partner; regaining sexual energy Wanting to feel creative, emotional, or sexual energy Performing or involved in inspirational activities Feeling abundance Engaging or expressing emotions with another person; for emotional balance; for strong positive emotional states Wanting to enhance clairsentience Playing with children Wanting to relax in solitude Watching movies Opening harmonious relationships with people

WHEN TO DIAL DOWN OR OPEN UP YOUR CHAKRAS

CHAKRA	DURING WHICH ACTIVITIES DO YOU DIAL DOWN THIS CHAKRA?	DURING WHICH ACTIVITIES DO YOU OPEN UP THIS CHAKRA?
3rd	Out of alignment with your sense of self; feeling willful, needy, nervous, anxious, doubtful, or panicky Wanting to maintain appropriate personal power and self-confidence Wanting to avoid power struggles or remain uninvolved Experiencing energy leaks or invasions Involved in conflict or negative situations or feeling too angry Involved in a consultation/meditation/healing Under stress or feeling financial concerns Wanting to maintain personal boundaries In the presence of skeptics or cynics Working Interacting with shy or extremely introverted persons In a crowd or group Wanting to concentrate the energies upward and have upper chakras more open and operating as the dominant receivers Wanting to go to sleep	Cleansing or clearing the chakra Involved in a consultation/meditation/healing Standing up for yourself, being in your power, improving relationship with yourself, exerting your will, or making a strong move in life Involved in conflict Wanting to enhance dream recall Wanting to enhance out-of-body experiences Feeling down or feeling personal power being drained Wanting to get a clear read on someone or something Wanting to be more alert or have more energy, strength, or vitality Staying focused or on task Wanting greater self-confidence, higher self-esteem, or greater internal strength; to enhance action and energy Claiming your own space, being more present, or standing up for your beliefs Wanting to feel carefree and joyful Promoting yourself; enhancing professional presence In negotiations Wanting increased creativity or improved performance

WHEN TO DIAL DOWN OR OPEN UP YOUR CHAKRAS

CHAKRA	DURING WHICH ACTIVITIES DO YOU DIAL DOWN THIS CHAKRA?	DURING WHICH ACTIVITIES DO YOU OPEN UP THIS CHAKRA?
4th	Feeling needy, insecure, overwhelmed, or emotional Overgiving or overly empathic Overly sentimental; feeling too much grief and pain (general bleeding-heart syndrome) Needing to take action on an intellectual level Experiencing energy invasions Creating boundaries or distance for emotional protection In hurtful situations or when susceptible to heartache Around untrustworthy people In threatening situations; when the environment is not loving and supportive Conducting business	Cleansing or clearing the chakra Involved in a consultation/ meditation/healing Expressing love, compassion, and forgiveness Tuning into emotional wisdom, confidence, and self-love Connecting in relationships or being more heart-focused Working with elders Around loved ones, children, or family Listening to music Accessing heart-centered creativity

	WHEN TO DIAL DOWN OR OPEN UP YOUR CHAKRAS	
CHAKRA	DURING WHICH ACTIVITIES DO YOU DIAL DOWN THIS CHAKRA?	DURING WHICH ACTIVITIES DO YOU OPEN UP THIS CHAKRA?
5th	Listening or allowing others to speak; receiving information during a conversation	Cleansing or clearing the chakra
		Involved in a consultation/ meditation/healing
	Feeling stifled by another spirit	Working with elders or children
	Needing to shield yourself from bullying	Wanting clear, direct, open, and balanced communication
	Fearing self-expression	Wanting to be more articulate or have greater self-expression
	Wanting to remain silent	
	Around judgmental people or authority figures	Speaking your truth
	Around overly egotistical people or people with confused energy	In social situations or professional situations/meetings; speaking in public
	Not wanting to overwhelm another during a conversation or a healing	Involved in creative activities or creative expression; to stimulate creativity
	Overtalking, overexplaining, or experiencing chatterbox syndrome	

	WHEN TO DIAL DOWN OR OPEN UP YOUR CHAKRAS	
CHAKRA	**DURING WHICH ACTIVITIES DO YOU DIAL DOWN THIS CHAKRA?**	**DURING WHICH ACTIVITIES DO YOU OPEN UP THIS CHAKRA?**
6th	Cleansing and clearing the chakra In meditation Feeling overwhelmed by too much information; overperceiving without the ability to discern what you are perceiving Wanting to turn down intuitive chatter or communication Wanting to avoid picking up too much intuitive information or knowledge Experiencing energy invasions Around too many intuitive people Wanting to calm, rest, and quiet the mind Around chaotic energy or stressful situations In crowds or around large groups of people Needing to go to sleep	Cleansing or clearing the chakra Involved in a consultation/ meditation/healing Wanting to get a clear perception of a person or situation Seeking clarity; wanting to perceive truth; solving problems Accessing or improving intuitive insight; wanting to increase perception, clairvoyance, inner knowing, second sight, revelation, or visions Accessing inner guidance or self-knowledge Around family Exploring the world of the mystic In nature Wanting to induce deep concentration Wanting to diminish an overanalyzing mind

	WHEN TO DIAL DOWN OR OPEN UP YOUR CHAKRAS	
CHAKRA	**DURING WHICH ACTIVITIES DO YOU DIAL DOWN THIS CHAKRA?**	**DURING WHICH ACTIVITIES DO YOU OPEN UP THIS CHAKRA?**
7th	In high-risk or dangerous activities Wanting to stay in the body Wanting to stay focused on the physical plane Feeling the body disconnected from the spirit Wanting to enhance strong grounding Wanting to go to sleep	Cleansing or clearing the chakra Involved in a consultation/meditation/healing Wanting to feel a spiritual connection or to connect with your higher self In dreams or revery or during prayer Accessing information on a universal or spiritual plane Wanting to diminish connection with the earth plane Wanting to leave the body

	WHEN TO DIAL DOWN OR OPEN UP YOUR CHAKRAS	
CHAKRA	**DURING WHICH ACTIVITIES DO YOU DIAL DOWN THIS CHAKRA?**	**DURING WHICH ACTIVITIES DO YOU OPEN UP THIS CHAKRA?**
Telepathic	Turning down intuitive chatter or communication Wanting to be completely present Tuning out other voices or other people's thoughts Entering into meditation; during meditation or healings Feeling headaches or facial tension Experiencing energy invasions Wanting to go to sleep; experiencing insomnia Wanting to avoid communication with people Under extreme stress Feeling you have done enough computer work for the day; after computer work In crowds or public places When the eyes and ears have taken in their maximum for the day	Cleansing or clearing the chakra Involved a consultation/meditation/healing Accessing or increasing intuition, knowing, or second sight Wanting to receive unspoken information or allow communication Wanting to increase perceptual awareness, discernment, and revelation Wanting to increase telepathy, clairvoyance, and clairaudience Desiring spirit-to-spirit communication Wanting to connect more deeply with others or "read" new people or situations Tuning into synchronicity Facilitating work communication Facilitating family relationships When scanning for danger signals in threatening or frightening situations

	WHEN TO DIAL DOWN OR OPEN UP YOUR CHAKRAS	
CHAKRA	DURING WHICH ACTIVITIES DO YOU DIAL DOWN THIS CHAKRA?	DURING WHICH ACTIVITIES DO YOU OPEN UP THIS CHAKRA?
Hand	Touching or around negative or aberrant energy Completing a healing or meditation Working on the computer; using a cell phone, other electronic devices, or digital media Involved in social events Working with kundalini energy Avoiding merging energies with other people Feeling too much energy running through the hands Under stress Hands feel too hot	Cleansing or clearing the chakra Involved in a consultation/ meditation/healing Accessing, receiving, or increasing incoming psychic vibrations or energy; working with psychometry; moving energy In prayer Giving and receiving love Hugging a person Accessing creativity Connecting to the earth Warming up hands or releasing stuck energy

WHEN TO DIAL DOWN OR OPEN UP YOUR CHAKRAS

CHAKRA	DURING WHICH ACTIVITIES DO YOU DIAL DOWN THIS CHAKRA?	DURING WHICH ACTIVITIES DO YOU OPEN UP THIS CHAKRA?
Feet	Other people are grounding through you Experiencing energy leaks or energy invasions Feet feel too hot or energy is not flowing into the feet and legs Needing energy protection or in threatening or frightening situations Wanting to astral-travel Feeling sleepy or lethargic	Cleansing or clearing the chakra Involved in a consultation/ meditation/healing Wanting to ground Feet are cold Wanting to circumvent altitude sickness or vertigo or to enhance balance Wanting to connect with earth energy

HOW DO YOU KNOW WHEN YOUR CHAKRAS ARE...

CHAKRA	IN HARMONY?	OUT OF HARMONY?
1st	Open, relaxed, grounded, heavy, balanced, rooted, sturdy, satisfied, capable, whole, centered, powerful, safe, confident, solid, stable, strong, and self-knowing Chakra has deep tones or earth tones; can feel the pulse of the earth, full and vibrant, rich and bright in color, flowing, and warm Fully present in the world and in present time; fully in the body; only personal energy is in the chakra Chakra has good rotation; full and round; spinning; at optimum resonance; actively working Invulnerable to other people's energy or invasion Devoted and responsible to spirit; open and harmonized with spirit	Ungrounded, troubles with basic life, confused, stressed, or in survival mode Fearful and self-doubting, anxious, irritable, insecure, sluggish, stiff, closed off from life, rigid, doubtful, suspicious, uneasy, or unbalanced Blocked, contracted, disconnected, uncomfortable, or stressed out Chakra not spinning correctly; feeling vacant or stagnant Chakra dark, dull, and dense, with no or little energy running through it; holes or smudges of energy interference Feeling like a volcano with energy roiling inside it Burning sensation in bladder area; back spasms; systemic (energetic, physical, and emotional) malfunctioning Cold, not present, "out of body," or "out of skin"

HOW DO YOU KNOW WHEN YOUR CHAKRAS ARE...		
CHAKRA	IN HARMONY?	OUT OF HARMONY?
2nd	Clear, smooth, vibrant, open, clean, healthy, happy, pure, grounded, renewed, centered, emotionally present, emotionally balanced, empowered, calm, soft yet strong, and pliable Creative, sexual, energetic, sensual, naturally empowered to manifest inspiration Chakra spinning, bright, dancing, alive, warm, energized, light, active, intact, and contained	Overstimulated olfactory sense Nymphomania/satyrism; sexual addiction Contracted, tight, grumpy, heavy, dark, bloated, unhappy, emotionally drained, unconfident, moody, emotionally needy, overly emotional, reactive, vulnerable, judgmental, overly empathic, ungrounded, numb, unfeeling, or emotionally distant Not emotionally present, not in present time, disconnected, or out of touch; difficulty in hearing inner voice Swings in sexuality or feeling unsexual; sexual dysfunction Butterflies in stomach, poor food choices, lower back pain, fatigue, lower intestinal disturbance, or feeling queasy Energy violations or drains; merged energy Chakra not spinning correctly

HOW DO YOU KNOW WHEN YOUR CHAKRAS ARE...

CHAKRA	IN HARMONY?	OUT OF HARMONY?
3rd	Vibrant, warm, empowered, and self-assured Confident, relaxed, energized, joyful, carefree, solid, strong, firm yet flexible, grounded, healthy, centered, powerful, settled, at ease, inwardly strong, calm, self-contained, and spirited Chakra shining, spinning, bright, and radiant Good digestion Able to know and recall astral activity In tune with personal power and self Cohesive social and community interactions	Punched-in-the-stomach feeling; butterflies in stomach, burning sensation in solar plexus, backache, food cravings, overeating, painful fiery burning, tight stomach, inability to breathe deeply, knot in stomach, or nausea Skin in the area is hot and hypersensitive to touch Powerless, disconnected, feelings of failure, imploded, overwhelmed, low self-esteem, defensive, irritable, fearful, inappropriate caretaking, ungrounded, stressed, dark, power struggles, feeling victimized, dominance issues, or low self-esteem Energy depleted, sleepy, lethargic, heavy, tired, exhausted, burned out, energetically invaded, or experiencing energetic struggles Nightmares; insomnia; difficulty waking up

HOW DO YOU KNOW WHEN YOUR CHAKRAS ARE...		
CHAKRA	IN HARMONY?	OUT OF HARMONY?
4th	Loving, kind, safe, alive, grounded, confident, centered, grateful, appreciative, patient, honoring self and others, balanced, open to giving and receiving love, empathic, generous, giving, nonjudgmental, open, relaxed, embracing, centered, whole, understanding, beautiful, loved, aware, lively, light, an lighthearted Creative and fulfilled Expansive, soft, fluid, warm, easy to open and close chakra, in alignment, in harmony, heart opening, alive, and chakra spinning Energetic boundaries, individuated, protected, and in personal heart space Compassionate, with discrimination	Unhappy, insecure, temperamental, closed, shut down, sad, not compassionate, ungrounded, impatient, emotionally guarded, despairing, grieving, emotionally disconnected, fearful, unloving, angry, frustrated, overly empathic, defended, suspicious of others' intentions, withholding, unloving, weighty, lacking energy, unlively, heartache, in emotional pain, emotionally hard, or overly giving Irregular heartbeat, false tachycardia, burning sensation in heart, cold-hearted, difficulty breathing or taking full breaths, shoulder or upper-back tension, slumped shoulders, defensive posture, or chest constricted Chakra has dark energy, and is not spinning correctly, shrunken, muted, or energetically entangled; energies are merged; blown out or blown open; boundaries violated

HOW DO YOU KNOW WHEN YOUR CHAKRAS ARE…		
CHAKRA	**IN HARMONY?**	**OUT OF HARMONY?**
5th	Communication and self-expression are free-flowing; open, caring, and passionate Grounded, creative, able to speak your mind, clear, confident, inspired, centered, vibrant, resonant, and relaxed Voice strong; inspired, expressive, and articulate; able to easily speak truth Empowered, dynamic, resourceful, laughing, liberated, and free Able to stand up for needs; communicative Clean, open, harmonized, responsive, chakra spinning, uninhibited, open, supple, and fluid as a song	Laryngitis or sore throat Crackly, hoarse voice Very quiet, unkind, uncreative, difficulty in expressing self, ungrounded, timid expression or communication, uninspired, inarticulate, overtalking, or talking over others Throat constriction, contraction, or tension Lump in throat, jaw tension, trouble swallowing, teeth-grinding, or throat clearing Dry, tight throat; thin breath; thin voice; vocal frustration Chakra closed, dark, or not spinning correctly; tight, choked or clogged, shut down, restricted, timid, or energetically blocked

HOW DO YOU KNOW WHEN YOUR CHAKRAS ARE...

CHAKRA	IN HARMONY?	OUT OF HARMONY?
6th	Open-minded, nonjudgmental, clear-thinking, peaceful, centered, grounded, receptive, lucid, and objective Insightful and intuitive Increased knowing and expanded perception Aware, open, empowered, resonant, and clairvoyant Extraordinary clarity in all perceptual systems; can clearly read between the lines of people's expressions, words, and body language Able to understand all animals and humans without analytical discussion Optimistic, powerful, stable, lucky, blessed, and mystically alive Relaxed face/forehead, soft eyes, and tingles in forehead In the moment, in present time, and experiencing synchronicity Chakra spinning, translucent, and crystalline	Inner light gone, acting stupid, excess energy, too many images, hallucinations, filtered perceptions, perceptually handicapped, limited, untrusting, or overanalyzing Limited or decreased perception, difficulty accessing intuitive information, unknowing, or clouded thinking Confusion, lack of clarity, subjectivity, or inability to utilize inner sight or knowing Headaches, eyestrain, eye discomfort, sinus problems, furrowed brow, tiredness, burning sensation in forehead, or pressure in head Disconnected from or difficulty connecting with spirit; loss of openness and spiritual creativity Chakra congested, dark, closed down, muddy, agitated, roiling, ungrounded, or not spinning correctly

HOW DO YOU KNOW WHEN YOUR CHAKRAS ARE...

CHAKRA	IN HARMONY?	OUT OF HARMONY?
7th	Aligned with higher self, grateful, or spiritually aware Chakras are aligned, harmonious, and there is a free-flowing circuit within energy systems; meditation is easy Strong sense of self, spirit, and spirituality Resonant, tingly, flowing, and connected to Universal Source Believing in the spiritual world Increased life force; feeling majestic; increased perception and strength of spirit Chakra symmetrical, firm, strong, capable of receiving universal energies, contained, spacious in an upward fashion, easy to open and close, sparkling, energetically alive, open, and aligned with spirit Grounded, present in body, in present time, centered, feeling self-worth and a balanced sense of self, open, secure, in harmony with your body and spirit, restful, calm, still, peaceful, resourceful, helpful, balanced, connected, and relaxed Warm, tingling feeling at crown	Craving sugar or alcohol; drug addiction Self-abuse Not trusting self, feeling alone, feeling worthless, or lacking self-respect Unconfident, out of body, not in present time, disconnected from spirit or the universe, not centered, ungrounded, restless, fatalistic, stuck inside head, spaced out, scared, discombobulated, painful, pressured, stupid, or martyrlike Pressure in head, tension in back of head and neck, atlas vertebrae out of line Chakra clogged, shallow, too open or hard to close, vulnerable to energetic violations, blown open, dark, not spinning correctly, or asymmetrical Questioning personal spirit and spirituality, diminished spiritual information, unable to sense life path, or spiritually disconnected

HOW DO YOU KNOW WHEN YOUR CHAKRAS ARE...		
CHAKRA	**IN HARMONY?**	**OUT OF HARMONY?**
Telepathic	Quiet and under control, alert, focused, able to gather information from environment, able to see and hear clearly, tuned in, able to send/receive information/energy successfully, able to sort out incoming chatter/energetic traffic, and communicating easily Chakra free, spinning, clear, bright, relaxed, and open Eyes soft, face relaxed, and mind quiet; no ringing in ears	Other voices inside head Head chatter, auditory bombardment/sensitivity, crazy thoughts, or looping conversations in head Unfocused, thoughts racing, agitated, excited and excitable, overwhelmed with stories, confused, distracted, or perception cloudy Indiscriminate mental chatter or inner perceptions; difficulty concentrating Tension around eyes, tension headache, sinus pressure, buzzing in head, ringing in ears Dark, foggy, clogged, pulsing, beating, or flickering; throbbing energy around eyes

HOW DO YOU KNOW WHEN YOUR CHAKRAS ARE...		
CHAKRA	IN HARMONY?	OUT OF HARMONY?
Hand	Sensitive, warm, open, creative, strong, powerful, tingly, sensing, aware, in control, conductive, and sensory Energy flowing freely, able to sense energies in people and things and send good energy, able to give and receive energy easily, healing energy flowing freely, and psychometry functioning well Chakra pulsating, expanded, open, flowing, rejuvenating, healing, and spinning Connected to your spirit; able to feel/sense spiritual energies Tinged with heat energy; tingly	Cramped, heavy, cold, or achy Insensitive, unresponsive, uncreative, numb, or manually clumsy Blocked energy, energy invasions, difficulty in moving or transmitting energy, unable to sense giving or receiving of energy, or loss of psychometric acuity Thick, sluggish, or clogged; unresponsive energy movement Pins and needles, inflamed, uncomfortably hot, throbbing, itching, dry, or pain in arms

HOW DO YOU KNOW WHEN YOUR CHAKRAS ARE...		
CHAKRA	IN HARMONY?	OUT OF HARMONY?
Feet	Grounded, connected to earth, warm, stable, secure, rooted, peaceful, balanced, safe, and calm Fully present in body Flowing, sensory, golden, open, pulsating, and full of energy Greater spiritual balance	Cramped, wobbly, disconnected, broken, cold, closed, tight, ungrounded, out of balance, constricted, or contracted Experiencing energetic leaks or trickling energy; unable to circulate energies Dull, achy, blockages and aches in legs, lack of sensation, stubbed toes, stiffness, or sciatica

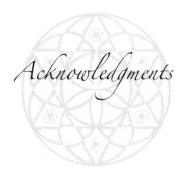

Acknowledgments

This book reflects not just my work but the efforts of many others. I would like to offer each of them my heartfelt thanks. Gina Vucci believed that this information deserved a wider audience and opened the door to my publisher, Nataraj Publishing/New World Library. I gave my manuscript to Shakti Gawain, who kindly accepted it and placed it at the bottom of a large pile of other manuscripts sitting on her desk, saying that it would be a while before she could find time to read it. Three days later, she phoned to say that my book was accepted for publication. Thank you, Shakti. The entire team at New World Library is exceptional. My editor, Georgia Hughes, was a master at seeing the "big picture" of my book and arranging the contents with clarity and style. Copyeditor Carol Venolia was a gifted wordsmith, contributing grounded questions and editorial suggestions about structure. Laura Harger was an exceptional proofreader. Elizabeth Rose Raphael brought all the elements of the book together with artistry and grace. Mary Ann Casler intuitively created the cover design, reflecting sketches I had done, before I had even described them to her. Designer Bill Mifsud created the inspired interior design, and production director Tona Pearce Myers oversaw the typesetting and design with attentiveness and care. Senior publicist Monique Muhlenkamp and marketing director Munro Magruder worked together as an invaluable team, blending business savvy with expert communication.

I am grateful to Christina Nelson, who designed accurate representational charts for the book based on my descriptions of energy anatomy. Thanks to Ian Sandiland for his original chart ideas, which we borrowed from my course-materials book, *Intuition Medicine: The Science of Energy*. I give blessings to the spirit of my computer for tirelessly working with me at all hours of the day and night in order to complete this book.

I offer a heartfelt thanks to all my students; your insights inspired me and your stories are the warp woven through this book. Many of you contributed creatively to this endeavor with your art, ideas and catalyzing words. You are the living books that I am honored to read. A short list of people who I thank for being in my life: Cecelia Vela Bailey, Warren Bellows, Theresa Biondo, Marlon and Pamela Bradley, Ken Choi, Jane Hogan, Ann Krcik, Theresa Lumiere, Amy Schaffer, Susie and Will Shipley, and Carol Spence.

I have been mentored by the writings, theory-challenging chats, and observations of people who examine concepts outside of the box. Some of the people who I admire for embodying their beliefs are Dick Blasband, Alan Charles, Larry Dossey, Bob Jahn, Dean Radin, Norm Shealy, Elisabeth Targ, Berney Williams, and Garret Yount.

The familial support of my brother, Ross Biondo, my husband, Michael McCartney, and our daughters, Zoe and Zena, weaves the fabric of love that holds me.

We are known by the communities in which we live, and I am proud to be a part of a collective of spirits who seek to know more about life and investigate all possibilities with compassion, humor, and open minds.

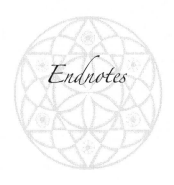

Endnotes

INTRODUCTION

Epigraph: Thich Nhat Hanh, *Living Buddha, Living Christ* (New York: Riverhead Books, 1995).

CHAPTER 2

Epigraph: Albert Einstein, quoted in *Bartlett's Familiar Quotations* (Boston: Little, Brown & Co., 1980).

1. *Random House College Dictionary,* 10th 5th ed., s.v. "intuition."
2. Ann T. McCluskey, "Intuition Medicine as an Effective Treatment in Psychiatric Nursing," *Journal of the Academy of Intuition Medicine* (March 2004), www.intuitionmedicine.com/journal/22journalnursingandim.htm.
3. Plotinus, *The Six Enneads* (Internet Classics Archive), http://classics.mit.edu/Plotinus/enneads.html.
4. Fritjof Capra, *The Tao of Physics* (Boston: Shambhala, 1975).
5. Diane Martindale, "The Body Electric," *New Scientist* (May 15, 2004): 35.
6. Carol Venolia, *Healing Environments* (Berkeley, Calif.: Celestial Arts, 1988).
7. Stephen Covey, *The 7 Habits of Highly Effective People* (New York: Fireside, 1998).

CHAPTER 3

Epigraph: Novalis, *The Novices of Sais* (New York: C. Valentine, 1949).

1. Francesca McCartney, "An Empirical Study of the Transmission of Healing Energy via E-mail," *International Journal of Healing and Caring — On-Line* (May 2004), www.ijhc.org.

2. Francesca McCartney, "The Conscious Internet: An Empirical Study of the Transmission of Healing Energy via E-mail," *Dynamical Psychology: An International, Interdisciplinary Journal of Complex Mental Processes,* (December 2003), www.goertzel.org/dynapsyc/2003/McCartney03.htm.
3. Francesca McCartney, "An Empirical Study of the Transmission of Healing Energy via E-mail."

CHAPTER 4

Epigraph: Mantak Chia, *The Inner Structure of Tai Chi* (Boston: Tuttle Publishing, 1998).
1. James Oschman, "Subtle Energies and Energy Medicine Instrumentation" (paper, International Society for the Study of Subtle Energy and Energy Medicine Annual Conference, Colorado Springs, Colo., June 27, 2004).
2. Eckhart Tolle, *The Power of Now* (Novato, Calif.: New World Library, 1999).
3. Trinity Sound Company, http://www.trinitysoundcompany.com.
4. The I Ching: Or Book of Changes (Princeton, N.J.: Princeton University Press, 1967).
5. Erich Fromm, *The Art of Loving* (New York: Perennial, 2000).
6. Dean Radin, *The Conscious Universe* (New York: HarperCollins, 1997), 174.
7. Judy Jacka, *The Vivaxis Connection* (Charlottesville, Va.: Hampton Roads Publishing, 2000), 70.
8. Ibid., xv–xvii.
9. James Oppenheim, *The Sea* (New York: Knopf, 1924).
10. Gwendolyn Bays, trans., *The Voice of the Buddha: The Beauty of Compassion* (Berkeley, Calif.: Dharma Publishing, 1983), 2:481–82.
11. Albert Einstein, *Ideas and Opinions* (New York: Crown, 1954).
12. Leonard Shlain, *Art and Physics: Parallel Visions in Space, Time, and Light* (New York: William Morrow, 1991), 353.
13. Arthur Zajonc, *Catching the Light* (New York: Bantam Books, 1993), 253.
14. Richard Gerber, *Vibrational Medicine* (Rochester, Vt.: Bear & Co., 2001), 524–25.
15. Corinne Heline, *Esoteric Music Based on the Musical Seership of Richard Wagner* (Los Angeles: New Age Press, 1953), 72.
16. Jack Schwarz, *Human Energy Systems* (New York: E. P. Dutton, 1980), 4.
17. Gerber, *Vibrational Medicine,* 520.

18. Michael Talbot, *The Holographic Universe* (New York: HarperPerennial, 1992), 292.
19. Steven Harnard, *Categorical Perception: The Groundwork of Cognition* (Cambridge: Cambridge University Press, 1987).
20. Chris Highland, ed., *Meditations of John Muir: Nature's Temple* (Berkeley, Calif.: Wilderness Press, 2001).

CHAPTER 5

Epigraph: Frances Vaughan, *Awakening Intuition* (New York: Anchor Books, 1979).

CHAPTER 6

Epigraph: Joseph Campbell, *The Mythic Image* (Princeton, N.J.: Princeton University Press, 1975).

1. Eckhart Tolle, *The Power of Now* (Novato, Calif.: New World Library, 1999), 110.
2. Albert Einstein, *Ideas and Opinions* (New York: Crown, 1954).
3. John Polkinghorne, *Faith, Science, & Understanding* (London and New Haven, Conn.: Yale University Press, 2000), 134–35.
4. Ray Villard, "Astrophysics Challenged by Dark Energy Finding," *Space.com* (April 10, 2001) www.space.com/scienceastronomy/ generalscience/darkenergy_folo_010410.html.
5. Stuart Clark, "Astronomers Detect the Universal Web," *New Scientist* (August 1, 2002) www.newscientist.com/article.ns?id=dn2624.
6. Itzhak Bentov, *A Brief Tour of Higher Consciousness* (Rochester, Vt.: Destiny Books, 2000), 43.
7. Candace Pert, *Molecules of Emotion* (New York: Scribner, 1997).
8. Brian Joseph Breiling, ed., *Light Years Ahead: Full Spectrum and Colored Light in Mindbody Healing* (Tiburon, Calif.: Light Years Ahead Publishing, 1996), 32–33.
9. Stanley Krippner and John White, *Future Science: Life Energies and the Physics of Paranormal Phenomena* (New York: Doubleday, 1977), 283.
10. Barbara Brennan, *Hands of Light* (New York: Bantam Books, 1988), 126.
11. Aldous Huxley, quoted in *Bartlett's Familiar Quotations* (Boston: Little, Brown & Co., 1980).
12. Julian Barbour, *The End of Time* (New York: Oxford University Press, 2000), 336–38.

13. Ibid., 16.

14. Ibid., 357.

15. Bentov, *A Brief Tour of Higher Consciousness,* 43.

16. Sharon Franquemont, *You Already Know What to Do* (New York: Tarcher/Putnam 1999), 163.

17. Lewis Carroll, *Alice in Wonderland* (New York: Norton & Co., 1989).

18. Olga Zharina, "Time Can Be Turned Back," *Pravda* (March 1, 2004) http://english.pravda.ru/science/19/94/379/12190_experiment.html.

19. Sheila Ostrander and Lynn Schroeder, *Psychic Discoveries behind the Iron Curtain* (New York: Bantam Books, 1973), 162–63.

20. Brennan, *Hands of Light,* 24.

21. Dean Radin, *The Conscious Universe* (New York: HarperCollins, 1997), 116.

22. Gwendolyn Bays, trans., *The Voice of the Buddha* (Berkeley, Calif.: Dharma Publishing, 1983).

23. Radin, *The Conscious Universe,* 279–81.

24. Michael Talbot, *The Holographic Universe* (New York: HarperPerennial, 1992), 226.

25. Andy and Larry Wachowski, *The Matrix,* DVD (Los Angeles: Warner Brothers Studios, 1999).

26. Robert Jahn, "Scientific Study of Consciousness-Related Physical Phenomena," Princeton Engineering Anomalies Research, www.princeton.edu/~pear/2.html.

27. Michael Brooks, "The Weirdest Link," *New Scientist* (March 27, 2004): 32–35.

28. Frances Vaughan, *Awakening Intuition* (New York: Anchor Books, 1979), 90.

29. Ibid., 185.

30. Dia North, *The Smart Spot* (Boston: Red Wheel/Weiser, 2003), 40.

31. Ibid., xiii.

32. Bays, *The Voice of the Buddha.*

33. Larry Dossey, "Standards in Healing Research: Working Definitions and Terms," *Alternative Therapies in Health and Medicine* (supplement) 9, no. 3 (Samueli Institute: Corona del Mar. *Alternative Therapies in Health and Medicine*: Supplement, Vol. 9, No.3, (2003): A11–A12.

34. William Tiller, "Healing Energy and Consciousness: Into the Future or a Retreat to the Past?" *Subtle Energies Journal* 5, no. 3 (1994): 254–55.

35. Arthur Zajonc, *Catching the Light* (New York: Bantam Books, 1993), 84.

36. W. C. Gough and R. L. Shacklett, "The Science of Connectiveness, Part III: The Human Experience," *Subtle Energies Journal* 4, no. 3 (1993): 208–09.
37. Brennan, *Hands of Light,* 126.
38. Nicholas Black Elk and John G. Neihardt, *Black Elk Speaks* (Lincoln, Neb.: University of Nebraska Press, 1988).
39. Carl Jung, *Synchronicity* (Princeton, N.J.: Princeton University Press, 1973).
40. Shakti Gawain, *Developing Intuition* (Novato, Calif.: Nataraj/New World Library, 2000).
41. Robert Jahn and Brenda Dunne, "Sensors, Filters, and the Source of Reality," *Journal of Scientific Exploration* 18, no. 4 (winter 2004): 11.
42. Marilyn Schlitz, "Child Spirit," *Shift Magazine,* no. 4 (September–November, 2004), 36.
43. N. A. Kozyrez, "On the Potential for Experimental Investigation of the Properties of Time" (a paper published in the Soviet Union in 1971).
44. William Tiller, *Science and Human Transformation: Subtle Energies, Intentionality and Consciousness* (Walnut Creek, Calif.: Paviour Publishing, 1997).

CHAPTER 7

Epigraph: Henry Miller, *A Literate Passion: Letters of Anaïs Nin and Henry Miller, 1932–1953* (New York: Harvest/HBJ Books, 1989).

CHAPTER 8

Epigraph: George Leonard, *The Silent Pulse* (East Rutherford, N.J.: Dutton, 1978).
1. Brian Greene, *The Elegant Universe* (New York: W. W. Norton, 1999), 14.
2. Trinh Xuan Thuan, *Chaos and Harmony: Perspectives on Scientific Revolutions of the Twentieth Century* (New York: Oxford University Press, 2001), 245.
3. Harold Saxton Burr, *Blueprint for Immortality* (London: C. W. Daniel Co., 1972), 127.
4. Mae-Wan Ho, "Assessing Food Quality by Its After-Glow," Institute of Science in Society (May 1, 2004) www.i-sis.org.uk/AFQFIA.php.
5. Richard Gerber, *Vibrational Medicine* (Rochester, Vt.: Bear & Co., 2001), 134–35.

6. Robert Becker, *The Body Electric: Electromagnetism and the Foundation of Life* (New York: William Morrow, 1998), 98.

7. Valerie Hunt, *Infinite Mind: Science of the Human Vibrations of Consciousness* (Malibu, Calif.: Malibu Publishing, 1996), 110–11.

8. Burr, *Blueprint for Immortality*, 124.

9. William Tiller, *Science and Human Transformation: Subtle Energies, Intentionality and Consciousness* (Walnut Creek, Calif.: Paviour Publishing, 1997), 180.

10. Gerber, *Vibrational Medicine*, 522–23.

11. Aleister Crowley, *Book of Thoth*, (York Beach, ME: Weiser Books, 1981).

12. Lynne McTaggart, *The Field: The Quest for the Secret of the Universe* (New York: HarperCollins, 2002), 21.

13. Tiller, *Science and Human Transformation*, 135.

14. McTaggart, *The Field*, 40.

15. Ibid., 50.

16. Len Saputo, *Prescriptions for Health*, radio program, KSET, San Francisco, (February 27, 2004).

17. Norman Shealy and Caroline Myss, "The Ring of Fire and DHEA: A Theory for Energetic Restoration of Adrenal Reserves," *Subtle Energies Journal* 6, no. 2 (1995): 169.

18. Lois Lindstrom, "The Light Stuff: Cold Laser Therapy Is Joining the Injury Treatment Team," *Washington Post*, February 17, 2004.

19. Walter Russell, *The Secret of Light* (Waynesboro, Va.: University of Science & Philosophy, 1974).

20. W. C. Gough and R. L. Shacklett, "The Science of Connectiveness, Part III: The Human Experience," *Subtle Energies Journal* 4, no. 3 (1993): 191.

21. Jacob Liberman, *Light: Medicine of the Future* (Santa Fe: Bear & Co., 1991), 158.

22. Matthew 5:14–16.

23. Itzhak Bentov, *Stalking the Wild Pendulum* (New York: E. P. Dutton, 1977), 30.

24. Gerber, *Vibrational Medicine*, 460.

25. The Future Force Foundation, *Health & Wellness: Natural Choices*, brochure, 1997.

26. Gerber, *Vibrational Medicine*, 529.

27. E. E. Richards, "Earth Rhythms," *Earth Resonance* (March 2004), http://home.gwi.net/~erichard/home.htm.

28. Kyoichi Nakagawa, MD, "Magnetic Field Deficiency Syndrome," *Japan Medical Journal* 2745 (December 4, 1976): 41.

29. Arne Groth, "Dowsing: Mathematical Harmony in the Solar System?" *The Global Oneness Commitment*, www.experiencefestival.com/a/Dowsing/id/2184.

30. The Beatles, "All You Need Is Love," from *Magical Mystery Tour*, Capitol B000002UDB, CD.

31. Gerber, *Vibrational Medicine*, 528.

32. Stanley Krippner and John White, *Future Science: Life Energies and the Physics of Paranormal Phenomena* (New York: Doubleday, 1977).

33. Hunt, *Infinite Mind*, 112.

34. Ibid., 200.

35. C. O. Mawson, ed., *Roget's Thesaurus* (New York: Rutherford, 1963).

36. Ralph Waldo Emerson, *Self-Reliance and Other Essays* (New York: Dover, 1993).

37. Frank Waters, *The Book of the Hopi* (New York: Penguin, 1977).

CHAPTER 9

Epigraph: Lao-tzu, *Wen-tzu* (Boston: Shambala, 1992).

CHAPTER 10

Epigraph: Alice A. Bailey, *A Treatise on White Magic* (New York: Lucis Publishing Co., 1951).

1. The *New Scientist* Staff, "Is This the Earliest Sign of Human Culture?" *New Scientist* (April 10, 2004): 8.

2. The International Swastika-Info Team, "Swastika — Hints and Signposts to the Origin of Mankind," *The Truth and Legend of the Swastika*, www.swastika-info.com.

3. Gwendolyn Bays, trans., *The Voice of the Buddha: The Beauty of Compassion* (Berkeley, Calif.: Dharma Publishing, 1983), 481.

4. William Blake, quoted in *Bartlett's Familiar Quotations* (Boston: Little, Brown & Co., 1980).

5. Lauren Artress, *Walking the Sacred Path: Rediscovering the Labyrinth as a Sacred Tool* (New York: Riverhead Books, 1996).

6. Candace Pert, *Molecules of Emotion* (New York: Scribner, 1997), 142–43.

7. Manly P. Hall, *The Secret Teachings of All Ages* (Los Angeles: Philosophical Research Society, 1975), CLXXXVI.

8. Sheila Ostrander and Lynn Schroeder, *Psychic Discoveries behind the Iron Curtain* (New York: Bantam Books, 1973), 227.

9. Stanley Krippner and John White, *Future Science: Life Energies and the Physics of Paranormal Phenomena* (New York: Doubleday, 1977), 222.

10. Richard Gerber, *Vibrational Medicine* (Rochester, Vt.: Bear & Co., 2001), 133.

11. Harold Saxton Burr, *Blueprint for Immortality* (London: C. W. Daniel Co., 1972), 103–05.

12. Joseph Campbell, *The Mythic Image* (Princeton, N.J.: Princeton University Press, 1975), 334.

13. Valerie Hunt, *Infinite Mind: Science of the Human Vibrations Consciousness* (Malibu, Calif.: Malibu Publishing, 1996), 214–15.

14. Harry S. Truman, quoted in *Bartlett's Familiar Quotations.*

15. John DeLuca and Ray Daly, "The Inner Alchemy of Buddhist Tantric Meditation," *Subtle Energies Journal* 13, no. 2 (2002): 201–02.

16. Marcel Proust, *In Search of Lost Time* (New York: Penguin, 2003).

17. William James, quoted in *Bartlett's Familiar Quotations* (Boston: Little, Brown & Co., 1980).

18. Adelle Davis, *Let's Eat Right to Keep Fit* (New York: Harcourt, 1970).

19. Len Saputo, *Boosting Immunity* (Novato, Calif.: New World Library, 2002).

CHAPTER 11

Epigraph: Manly P. Hall, *The Secret Teachings of All Ages* (Los Angeles: Philosophical Research Society, 1975).

CHAPTER 12

Epigraph: Manly P. Hall, *Paracelsus, His Mystical and Medical Philosophy* (Los Angeles: Philosophical Research Society, 1990).

1. Harold Saxton Burr, *Blueprint for Immortality* (London: C. W. Daniel Co., 1972).

2. Richard Gerber, *Vibrational Medicine* (Rochester, Vt.: Bear & Co., 2001), 133–34.

3. William Tiller, *Science and Human Transformation: Subtle Energies, Intentionality, and Consciousness* (Walnut Creek, Calif.: Paviour Publishing, 1997), 107.

4. Ibid., 128.

5. Matthew 6:22 (King James Version).

6. Novalis, *The Novices of Sais* (New York: C. Valentine, 1949).

7. Edgar Cayce, *Auras* (Virginia Beach, Va.: A.R.E. Press, 2003).

8. Chinese aphorism, *All Spirit,* www.allspirit.co.uk/index.html.

9. David Tansley, *Radionics and the Subtle Anatomy of Man* (London: Straker Brothers Ltd., 1974), 17.

10. Albert Einstein, quoted in *Bartlett's Familiar Quotations* (Boston: Little, Brown & Co., 1980).

11. Robert Becker, *The Body Electric: Electromagnetism and the Foundation of Life* (New York: William Morrow, 1998).

12. Rudolph Steiner, *Truth-Wrought Words* (Spring Valley, N.Y.: Anthroposophic Press, 1979).

13. Lao-tzu, *Wen-tzu* (Boston: Shambala, 1992).

CHAPTER 13

Epigraph: J. B. von Helmont cited by Manly P. Hall, *The Secret Teachings of All Ages* (Los Angeles: Philosophical Research Society, 1975).

CHAPTER 14

Epigraph: Oscar Wilde, *Oscar Wilde's Wit and Wisdom* (New York: Dover, 1998).

1. Leonard Shlain, *Art and Physics: Parallel Visions in Space, Time, and Light* (New York: William Morrow, 1991), 171.

2. John Russell, *Matisse: Father and Son* (New York: Harry N. Abrams, 1999).

3. Leatrice Eiseman, *Colors for Your Every Mood* (Sterling, Va.: Capitol Books, 1998), 8.

4. Shlain, *Art and Physics,* 176–79.

5. Hunt, *Infinite Mind: Science of the Human Vibrations of Consciousness* (Malibu, Calif.: Malibu Publishing, 1960), 315–17.

6. Zajonc, *Catching the Light* (New York: Bantam Books, 1993), 5–15.

7. Robert Jahn and Brenda Dunne, "Sensors, Filters, and the Source of Reality," *Journal of Scientific Exploration* 18, no. 4 (winter 2004): 11.

8. Leatrice Eiseman and Lawrence Herbert, *The Book of Color* (New York: Harry N. Abrams, 1990), 9.

9. Philip Ross, "Insights: Draining the Language Out of Color," *Scientific American* (April 2004): 47.

10. Trevor Lamb, ed., *Colour, Art & Science* (Cambridge: Cambridge University Press, 1999), 6.

11. Eiseman, *Colors for Your Every Mood,* 8.

12. Hunt, *Infinite Mind,* 318.

13. Charles Klotsche, *Color Medicine* (Sedona, Ariz.: Light Technology Publishing, 1993), 46.

14. Roger Lewis, quoted in *Bartlett's Familiar Quotations* (Boston: Little, Brown & Co., 1980).

15. Jacob Liberman, *Light: Medicine of the Future* (Santa Fe: Bear & Co., 1991), 158.
16. Ibid., 158–59.
17. Zajonc, *Catching the Light*, 84.
18. Lamb, *Colour, Art & Science*, 104.
19. James Oschman, *Energy Medicine: The Scientific Basis* (London: Churchill Livingstone, 2003), 182.
20. Lamb, *Colour, Art & Science*, 138–39.
21. Pablo Picasso, *Picasso Erotique* (London: Prestel Publishing, 2001).
22. Lamb, *Colour, Art & Science*, 123–25.
23. Barbara Bowers, *What Color Is Your Aura?* (New York: Pocket Books, 1989), 10.
24. David Servan-Schreiber, *The Instinct to Heal: Curing Stress, Anxiety, and Depression Without Drugs and Without Talk Therapy* (New York: Rodale Press, 2004), 107.
25. Katherine Creath, "Measuring Effects of Healing Energy on Plant Leaves Using Biophoton Imaging" (paper, International Society of Subtle Energies and Energy Medicine Annual Conference, Colorado Springs, Colo., June 27, 2004).
26. Oschman, *Energy Medicine*, 88.
27. Daniel Benor, *Healing Research* (Medford, N.J.: Wholistic Healing Publications, 2004), vol. 2, 406.
28. Walt Whitman, *Walt Whitman: The Complete Poems*, ed. Francis Murphy (New York: Penguin Books, 1990), 127.
29. Alison Motluk, "How Minds Play Tricks with Words and Colours," *New Scientist* (August 21–27, 2004): 9.
30. Bruce Durie, "Why You Have at Least 21 Senses," *New Scientist* (January 29–February 4, 2005): 33–43.
31. Gabriel Cousins, MD, *Spiritual Nutrition and the Rainbow Diet* (Boulder, Colo.: Cassandra Press, 1987).
32. Alan Charles and Francesca McCartney, "The Effects of Energy and Color in Health and Behavior" (paper, International Academy of Preventive Medicine Annual Conference, Denver, 1980).
33. Betty Wood, *Healing Power of Color* (Rochester, Vt.: Destiny Books, 1998), 30.
34. C. J. Sander, *Practical Numerology and Character Analysis* (Whitefish, Mont.: Kessinger Publishing, 2003).

35. Oschman, *Energy Medicine*, 96.
36. Belleruth Naparstek, *Your Sixth Sense* (San Francisco: HarperSanFrancisco, 1997), 10.
37. Edvard Munch, on his painting "The Scream", *The Oxford Dictionary of Quotations* (Oxford: Oxford University Press, 1995).
38. Edgar Cayce, *Color,* (Virginia Beach, Va.: A.R.E. Press, 2004).
39. John Ruskin, *Lectures on Art* (New York: Allworth Press, 1996).

CHAPTER 15

Epigraph: Johann Wolfgang von Goethe, *Faust I & II* (Princeton, N.J.: Princeton University Press, 1994).

AFTERWORD

Epigraph: Norman Shealy and Caroline Myss, *The Creation of Health* (Walpole, N.H.: Stillpoint Press, 1988).

APPENDIX 1

Epigraph: Manly P. Hall, *Paracelsus, His Mystical and Medical Philosophy* (Los Angeles: Philosophical Research Society, 1990).

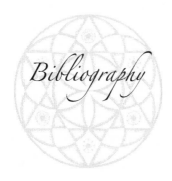

Bibliography

Aczel, Amir. *Entanglement*. New York: Four Walls Eight Windows, 2002.

Allen, James. *As a Man Thinketh*. Marina del Rey, Calif.: DeVorss & Company, 1983.

Andrews, Ted. *How to Heal with Color*. St. Paul, Minn.: Llewellyn Publications, 2001.

Barbour, Julian. *The End of Time*. New York: Oxford University Press, 2000.

Bays, Gwendolyn, trans. *The Voice of the Buddha: The Beauty of Compassion*. No. 2. Berkeley, Calif.: Dharma Publishing, 1983.

Becker, Robert. *The Body Electric: Electromagnetism and the Foundation of Life*. New York: William Morrow, 1998.

Benor, Daniel. *Spiritual Healing*. Vol. 1. Southfield, Mich.: Vision Publications, 2001.

———. *Healing Research*. Vol. 2. Medford, N.J.: Wholistic Healing Publications, 2004.

Bentov, Itzhak. *Stalking the Wild Pendulum*. New York: E. P. Dutton, 1977.

———. *A Brief Tour of Higher Consciousness*. Rochester, Vt.: Destiny Books, 2000.

Berger, Ruth. *The Secret Is in the Rainbow*. York Beach, Calif: Samuel Weiser, 1986.

Besant, Annie, and Leadbeater, C. W. *Thought-Forms*. Wheaton, Ill.: Theosophical Publishing House, 1969.

Birren, Faber. *Color in Your World*. New York: Macmillan Publishing Company, 1979.

Bowers, Barbara. *What Color Is Your Aura?* New York: Pocket Books, 1989.

Breiling, Brian Joseph, ed. *Light Years Ahead: Full Spectrum and Colored Light in Mindbody Healing.* Tiburon, Calif.: Light Years Ahead Publishing, 1996.

Brennan, Barbara. *Hands of Light.* New York: Bantam Books, 1988.

―――. *Light Emerging.* New York: Bantam Books, 1993.

Brown, Jason. *Mind, Brain and Consciousness.* New York: Academic Press, 1977.

Bruyere, Rosalyn. *Wheels of Light.* New York: Fireside Book, 1994.

Burr, Harold Saxton. *Blueprint for Immortality.* London: C. W. Daniel Co., 1972.

Campbell, Joseph. *The Mythic Image.* Princeton, N.J.: Princeton University Press, 1975.

Capra, Fritjof. *The Tao of Physics.* Boston: Shambhala, 1975.

Cardena, Etzel, ed. *Varieties of Anomalous Experience: Examining the Scientific Evidence.* Washington, D.C.: American Psychological Association, 2000.

Cayce, Edgar. *Auras.* Virginia Beach, Va.: A.R.E. Press, 2003.

―――. *Color.* Virginia Beach, Va.: A.R.E. Press, 2004.

Charles, Alan, and Francesca McCartney. "The Effects of Energy and Color in Health and Behavior." Paper, International Academy of Preventive Medicine Annual Conference, Denver, Colo., 1980.

Choi, C. "Biophoton Emission from the Hands." *Journal of the Korean Physical Society* 41, no. 2 (2002): 275–78.

Chopra, Deepak. *How to Know God.* New York: Harmony Books, 2000.

―――. *The Spontaneous Fulfillment of Desire.* New York: Harmony Books, 2003.

Coelho, Paulo. *The Alchemist.* New York: HarperCollins, 1988.

Cohen, S., and F. A. Popp. "Biophoton Emission of the Human Body." *Journal of Photochemistry and Photobiology* 40 (1997).

Cole, K. C. *Sympathetic Vibrations.* New York: Bantam Books, 1984.

Creath, Katherine. "Measuring Effects of Healing Energy on Plant Leaves Using Biophoton Imaging." Paper, International Society of Subtle Energies and Energy Medicine Annual Conference, Colorado Springs, Colo., June 27, 2004.

DeLuca, John, and Ray Daly. "The Inner Alchemy of Buddhist Tantric Meditation." *Subtle Energies Journal* 13, no. 2 (2002).

Dossey, Larry. *Reinventing Medicine.* San Francisco: HarperSanFrancisco, 1997.

―――. *Healing Words.* New York: HarperCollins, 1999.

―――. "Standards in Healing Research: Working Definitions and Terms." *Alternative Therapies in Health and Medicine* 9, no. 3, supplement (2003).

Eiseman, Leatrice. *The PANTONE Book of Color.* New York: Times Mirror, 1990.

―――. *Colors for Your Every Mood.* Sterling, Va.: Capitol Books, 1998.

Emery, Marcia. *The Intuitive Healer.* New York: St. Martin's Press, 1999.

Franquemont, Sharon. *You Already Know What to Do*. New York: Tarcher/ Putnam, 1999.

Ferrer, Jorge. *Revisioning Transpersonal Theory*. Albany, NY: State University of New York Press, 2002.

The Future Force Foundation. *Health & Wellness: Natural Choices*. Brochure, 1997.

Gawain, Shakti. *Developing Intuition*. Novato, Calif.: Nataraj/New World Library, 2000.

———. *Creative Visualization*. Novato, Calif.: Nataraj/New World Library, 2002.

Gerber, Richard. *Vibrational Medicine*. Rochester, Vt.: Bear & Co., 2001.

Gladwell, Malcolm. *Blink*. New York: Little, Brown and Co., 2005.

Goldman, Caren, "Intuitive Wisdom in the Laboratory." *Intuition Magazine* (June 1998): 21–25.

Goldner, Diane. *Infinite Grace*. Virginia Beach, Va.: Hampton Roads Publishing, 1999.

Gough, W. C., and R. L. Shacklett. "The Science of Connectiveness, Part III: The Human Experience." *Subtle Energies Journal* 4, no. 3 (1993).

Grad, Bernard. "The Biological Effects of the 'Laying on of Hands' on Animals and Plants: Implications for Biology." Chap. 10 in *Parapsychology: Its Relation to Physics, Biology, Psychology and Psychiatry*. Medford, N.J.: Scarecrow Press, 1976.

Green, Elmer. *The Ozawkie Book of the Dead*. Los Angeles: Philosophical Research Society, 2001.

Greene, Brian. *The Elegant Universe*. New York: W. W. Norton, 1999.

———. *The Fabric of the Cosmos*. New York: Random House, 2004.

Grof, Stanislav. *The Holotropic Mind*. San Francisco: HarperSanFrancisco, 1990.

Hall, Manly P. *The Secret Teachings of All Ages*. Los Angeles: The Philosophical Research Society, 1975.

Hawking, Stephen. *A Brief History of Time*. New York: Bantam Books, 1988.

———. *The Universe in a Nutshell*. New York: Bantam Books, 2001.

Heline, Corinne. *Esoteric Music Based on the Musical Seership of Richard Wagner*. Los Angeles: New Age Press, 1953.

Hoffman, Enid. *Develop Your Psychic Skills*. Rockport, Conn.: Para Research, 1981.

The Holy Bible. King James Version. Kansas City, Mo.: National Publishing Co., 1979.

Hunt, Roland. *The Seven Keys to Colour Healing*. London: C. W. Daniel Co., 1958.

Hunt, Valerie. *Infinite Mind: Science of the Human Vibrations of Consciousness.* Malibu, Calif.: Malibu Publishing, 1996.

Jacka, Judy. *The Vivaxis Connection.* Charlottesville, Va.: Hampton Roads Publishing, 2000.

Jahn, Robert, and Brenda Dunne. *Margins of Reality.* Orlando, Fla.: Harcourt Brace & Co., 1987.

———. "Sensors, Filters, and the Source of Reality." *Journal of Scientific Exploration* 18, no. 4 (Winter 2004).

Khavari, Khalil. *Spiritual Intelligence: A Practical Guide to Personal Happiness.* New Liskeard, Can.: White Mountain Publications, 2000.

Klotsche, Charles. *Color Medicine.* Sedona, Ariz.: Light Technology Publishing, 1993.

Krippner, Stanley, and John White. *Future Science: Life Energies and the Physics of Paranormal Phenomena.* New York: Doubleday, 1977.

Lamb, Trevor, ed. *Colour, Art & Science.* Cambridge: Cambridge University Press, 1999.

Leadbeater, C. W. *The Chakras.* Wheaton, Ill.: Theosophical Publishing House, 1974.

Lederman, Leo. *The God Particle.* New York: Delta Books, 1993.

LeShan, Lawrence. *The Medium, the Mystic, and the Physicist.* New York: Viking Press, 1974.

Liberman, Jacob. *Light: Medicine of the Future.* Santa Fe: Bear & Co., 1991.

Libet, Benjamin, ed. *The Volitional Brain.* Exeter, UK: Imprint Academic, 1999.

Lindgren, C. E., ed. *Capturing the Aura.* Nevada City, Calif.: Blue Dolphin Publishing, 2000.

Lindstrom, Lois. "The Light Stuff: Cold Laser Therapy Is Joining the Injury Treatment Team." *Washington Post,* February 17, 2004.

McCartney, Francesca. *The Intentional Encapsulation of Healing Energy and Its Transmission over the Internet.* Unpublished doctoral dissertation, Greenwich University, Australia, 2002.

McTaggart, Lynne. *The Field: The Quest for the Secret of the Universe.* New York: HarperCollins, 2002.

Motluk, Alison. "How Minds Play Tricks with Words and Colours." *New Scientist* (August 21–27, 2004).

Murphy, Michael. *The Future of the Body.* New York: Tarcher/Putnam, 1999.

Myss, Caroline. *Anatomy of the Spirit.* New York: Random House, 1996.

Nakagawa, Kyoichi. *Japan Medical Journal* 2745 (December 4, 1976).

Naparstek, Belleruth. *Your Sixth Sense*. San Francisco: HarperSanFrancisco, 1997.

Newberg, Andrew and Eugene D'Aquili. *Why God Won't Go Away*. New York: Ballantine, 2001.

Newton, Michael. *Journey of Souls*. St. Paul, Minn.: Llewellyn Publications, 1998.

North, Dia. *The Smart Spot*. Boston: Red Wheel/Weiser, 2003.

Orloff, Judith. *Second Sight*. New York: Warner Books, 1996.

———. *Positive Energy*. New York: Warner Books, 2004.

Oschman, James. *Energy Medicine: The Scientific Basis*. London: Churchill Livingstone, 2003.

———. "Subtle Energies and Energy Medicine Instrumentation." Paper, International Society of Subtle Energies and Energy Medicine Annual Conference, Colorado Springs, Colo., June 27, 2004.

Oslie, Pamala. *Life Colors*. Novato, Calif.: New World Library, 2000.

Ostrander, Sheila, and Lynn Schroeder. *Psychic Discoveries behind the Iron Curtain*. New York: Bantam Books, 1973.

Pert, Candace. *Molecules of Emotion*. New York: Scribner, 1997.

Pinker, Steve. *How the Mind Works*. New York: W. W. Norton, 1997.

Polkinghorne, John. *Faith, Science & Understanding*. London and New Haven, Conn.: Yale University Press, 2000.

Powell, Arthur. *The Causal Body*. Wheaton, Ill.: Theosophical Publishing House, 1956.

———. *The Mental Body*. Wheaton, Ill.: Theosophical Publishing House, 1956.

———. *The Solar System*. Wheaton, Ill.: Theosophical Publishing House, 1957.

Radin, Dean. *The Conscious Universe*. New York: HarperCollins, 1997.

Ramachandran, Vilayanur. "Hearing Colors, Tasting Shapes." *Scientific American* (May 2003): 53–59.

Rector-Page, Linda. *Healthy Healing*. Sacramento, Calif.: Spilman, 1990.

Regush, Nicholas. *The Human Aura*. New York: Berkeley Publishing Co., 1974.

Ross, Philip. "Draining the Language Out of Color." *Scientific American* (April 2004): 46–47.

Saputo, Len. "Prescriptions for Health." Radio program, KSET, San Francisco (February 27, 2004).

Satinover, Jeffrey. *The Quantum Brain*. New York: John Wiley & Sons, 2001.

Schlitz, Marilyn. "Child Spirit." *Shift Magazine* 4 (September–November 2004): 36.

Schlitz, Marilyn, and Tina Amorok. *Consciousness & Healing*. St. Louis: Elsevier Churchill Livingstone, 2005.

Schul, Bill. *The Psychic Frontiers of Medicine*. Greenwich, Conn.: Fawcett Publications, 1977.

Schultz, Mona Lisa. *Awakening Intuition*. New York: Harmony Books, 1998.

Schwarz, Jack. *Human Energy Systems*. New York: E. P. Dutton, 1980.

Servan-Schreiber, David. *The Instinct to Heal: Curing Stress, Anxiety, and Depression Without Drugs and Without Talk Therapy*. New York: Rodale Press, 2004.

Sexson, Mark. *The Power of Color*. Boston: Christopher Publishing House, 1938.

Shealy, Norman, and Caroline Myss. *The Creation of Health*. Walpole, N.H.: Stillpoint Press, 1988.

———. "The Ring of Fire and DHEA: A Theory for Energetic Restoration of Adrenal Reserves." *Subtle Energies Journal* 6, no. 2 (1995).

Sheldrake, Rupert. *The Sense of Being Stared At*. New York: Three Rivers Press, 2004.

Shlain, Leonard. *Art and Physics: Parallel Visions in Space, Time, and Light*. New York: William Morrow, 1991.

———. *The Alphabet and the Goddess*. New York: William Morrow, 2002.

Sui, Choa Kok. *Advanced Pranic Healing*. Chino, Calif.: Institute for Inner Studies, 2000.

Swanson, Claude. *The Synchronized Universe*. Tucson. Ariz.: Poseidia Press, 2003.

Talbot, Michael. *The Holographic Universe*. New York: HarperPerennial, 1992.

Tansley, David. *Radionics and the Subtle Anatomy of Man*. London: Straker Brothers Ltd., 1974.

Thuan, Trinh Xuan. *Chaos and Harmony: Perspectives on Scientific Revolutions of the Twentieth Century*. New York: Oxford University Press, 2001.

Tiller, William. "Healing Energy and Consciousness: Into the Future or a Retreat to the Past?" *Subtle Energies Journal* 5, no. 3 (1994).

———. *Science and Human Transformation: Subtle Energies, Intentionality and Consciousness*. Walnut Creek, Calif.: Paviour Publishing, 1997.

Tiller, William, Walter Dibble, and Michael Kohane. *Conscious Acts of Creation*. Walnut Creek, Calif.: Paviour Publishing, 2001.

Tolle, Eckhart. *The Power of Now.* Novato, Calif.: New World Library, 1999.

———. *Stillness Speaks.* Novato, Calif.: New World Library, 2003.

Twicken, David. *Spiritual Qi Gong.* Lincoln, Neb.: Author's Choice Press, 2001.

Vaughan, Frances. *Awakening Intuition.* New York: Anchor Books, 1979.

Verner-Bonds, Lillian. *Color Healing.* New York: Sterling Publishing, 2000.

Waechter, Randall, and Lauren Sergio. "Manipulation of the Electromagnetic Spectrum via Fields Projected from Human Hands." *Subtle Energies Journal* 13, no. 3 (2002): 9.

Westlake, Aubrey. *The Pattern of Health.* Berkeley, Calif.: Shambhala, 1973.

Whiting, Sam. "More Than Medicine." *San Francisco Chronicle Alternative Medicine Magazine* (June 6, 2004): 9.

Wood, Betty. *Healing Power of Color.* Rochester, Vt.: Destiny Books, 1998.

Yeffeth, Glenn, ed. *Taking the Red Pill.* Dallas, Tex.: Benbella Books, 2003.

Yount, Garret. "Biofield Perception: A Series of Pilot Studies with Cultured Human Cells." *Journal of Alternative and Complementary Medicine* 10, no. 3 (2004): 9.

Zajonc, Arthur. *Catching the Light.* New York: Bantam Books, 1993.

WEBSITES

Benor, Daniel, ed. *The International Journal of Healing and Caring.*
www.ijhc.org.
Brukner, Caslav. "Quantum Entanglement in Time." Blackett Laboratory,
Imperial College, London (February 2004), www.arxiv.org/abs/quant-
ph/0402127.
Davis, Cynthia. "Mindwise." *Mindwise* (February 2004) www.mindwise.com.au/
spiritual_intelligence.shtm.
Farrow, Kevin. "Some Notes on Working with Chakra Energies and Energy
Balancing." *Kheper* (April 2004) www.kheper.net/topics/chakras/
balancing.html.
Groth, Arne. "Dowsing: Mathematical Harmony in the Solar System?" *Dowsing*
(March 2004), www.experiencefestival.com/index.php/topic/articles/
article/2184.
Kurtus, Ron. "Modern Views of the Force of Gravity." *Kurtus School of
Champions* (February 2003), www.school-for-champions.com/science/
forcedistance.htm.
McCartney, Francesca. "The Conscious Internet: An Empirical Study of the
Transmission of Healing Energy via E-mail." *Dynamical Psychology: An
International, Interdisciplinary Journal of Complex Mental Processes*
(December 2003), www.goertzel.org/dynapsyc/dynacon.html.
———. "An Empirical Study of the Transmission of Healing Energy via
E-mail." *International Journal of Healing and Caring — On Line* (May,
2004), www.ijhc.org.
McCluskey, Ann T. "Intuition Medicine as an Effective Treatment in Psychiatric
Nursing." *Journal of the Academy of Intuition Medicine* (March 2004),
www.intuitionmedicine.com/journal/22journalnursingandim.htm.
Richards, E. E. "Earth Rhythms." *Earth Resonance* (March 2004),
http://home.gwi.net/~erichard/home.htm.
Villard, Ray. "Astrophysics Challenged by Dark Energy Finding." (2001,
April) Retrieved from: Space.com. www.space.com/scienceastronomy/
generalscience/darkenergy_folo_010410.html
———. "Astronomers Detect the Universal Web." (2002, August) Retrieved
from: New Scientist.com archives. www.newscientist.com.

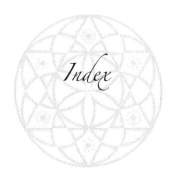

Index

Note: Page numbers in *italics* refer to illustrations.

A

Academy of Eastern Medicine (Walnut Creek, Calif.), 18–19, 227
Academy of Intuition Medicine (San Francisco Bay Area), 19, 33–34, 247
acupuncture, 18–19, 116, 154–55, 190
adrenal glands, 143, 146
affirmations
    aura, 209–10
    chakra, 175
    color, 242
    in daily use, 246
    earth-energy, 139
    grounding, 69–70
    life-force energy, 139
    meditation-sanctuary, 87, 104
    overview, 6
alchemy, medieval, 110

anamnesis (soul's remembrance of truth), 85
anamorphosis, 181
anger, repressed, 83
ani (aura), 180
animal magnetism, 110
antioxidants, 39
archaeus (life force), 109
assessing intuitive abilities, 8, 31–37
astral body/light, 180, 181
atomic structure, 213
atua (aura), 180
auras, 177–210
    affirmations for, 209–10
    awareness of, 195–96
    clairvoyant/clairaudient perception of, 177–78, 187
    colors of, 178, 183, 213, 218
    in daily life, 191–94, 208–9
    depictions of/names for, 180–81
    diagnosis and healing practice, 205
    diagnosis of energy of, 206–7
    disease detected via, 179, 188–89

auras (*continued*)
and the electric body of health, 190–91
energy collected in/broadcast by, 189
enhancing/depleting, 198–99
grounded, 179
grounding via, 40, *41*
healing of, 205–7, 209–10
health issues reference chart, 251–52, 254
healthy, benefits of, 196–98
healthy, characteristics of, 178
Kirlian, 181
layers/sheaths of, 181, 182, 183–84, 184–86, 187–88, 206
life-force energy as creating, 180–81
meditation/healing practice, 194–95, 201–2, 203, 204–10
as networks for subtle energies, 178–79
observational practices, 207–8
overview, 9
perspectives on the auric field, 188–89
as a protective energy skin, 177–78, 179, 191–93
reflections (exercise), 196–98
sensing of, 186–88
shapes of, 178
symbolism of, 180
and trust, 210
as a universally accepted phenomenon, 180–81
visualizations of, 193–94

aureoles, 180
awareness, intuitive, 7
of auras, 195–96
of color health needs, 232–35
indications of, 21–29
research, 33–36
ayik (aura), 180

B

Balinese religion, 142
baraka (life force), 109
Bhagavad Gita, 12
Bio-Acoustics healing, 108–9
bio-cosmic energy, 110
bioelectric fields, 27, 181
biofeedback machines, 27
bioluminescence, 181
biomagnetism, 110
biophotons, 187
bioplasma, 181
Body of Health, suggestions for use, 245–47
Bohm, David, 217
Boyle, Robert, 212
Brennan, Barbara, 74, 82
Bruyere, Rosalyn, 183
Buddha, 50, 142

C

California Pacific Medical Center (San Francisco), 23
Catholic-occultism, 11–12
causal body, 181
cause and effect, 80
chakra(s), 141–76
affirmations for, 175

aura layers generated by, 181, *182*,
    183–84, 187
colors of, 159, 161–62
contemplative meditations,
    161–62, 167–68
in daily life, 160–61, 174
definitions, 144, *145–46*, 147–49,
    159–60
electrical currents through, 152
and endocrine glands, 143–44,
    146, 152–53, 183
energy-transmisson of, 8, 152–54
enhancing/depleting, 165–66
fifth, 121, 143, *145–46*, 147–48,
    262, 272
fourth, 143, *145–46*, 147, 261, 271
grounding meditation, 168–70
grounding via, 40, *41*
harmony of, 268–77
and health, 154–56, 163–64
health issues reference chart,
    251–52, 254
journaling (exercise), 163–64
life-force and earth-energy medi-
    tation, 170–74
life-force energy in, 155–56
locations, 143–44, *145–46*
model for workings of, 150–52
and music, 53
openness of (dialing up/down),
    151, 159, 160–61, 170,
    257–67
other names for, 157
reference charts, 9
reflections (exercise), 163–64
sacred science of, 156–57
second, 143, *145–46*, 147, 259–60
seven's symbolism, 153
seventh, 121, 143, *145–46*, 148,
    264, 274
sixth, 91, 143, *145–46*, 148, 263,
    273
size of, 151
spin of, 151–52
symbolism/meaning of, 141–42,
    157
third, 143, *145–46*, 147, 260, 270
as three-dimensional, 149–50
and trust, 176
visualization/imagination in
    meditation, 158
wisdom wheels, 159–60
See also chakra reference charts;
    feet chakras; first chakra;
    hand chakras; telepathic
    chakras
chakra reference charts, 257–77
    dialing up/down, 258–67
    feet chakras, 267, 277
    fifth chakra, 262, 272
    first chakra, 258, 268
    fourth chakra, 261, 271
    hand chakras, 266, 276
    harmony, 268–77
    second chakra, 259, 269
    seventh chakra, 264, 274
    sixth chakra, 263, 273
    telepathic chakras, 265, 275
    third chakra, 260, 270
charisma, 208–9
Charles, Alan, 18–19
chi (life force), 109
children's grounding, 54–56
Chinese medicine. *See* acupuncture
chromotherapy, 227
circles of light, 157

clairaudience
  assessment, 32–33
  author's personal experiences, 13,
    17, 89
  characterization of, 24
clairsentience
  assessment, 32–33, 36
  characterization of, 24
  grounding via, 54
clairvoyance
  assessment, 32–33
  auras perceived via, 177–78, 187
  author's personal experiences, 13,
    18–19, 224–25
  characterization of, 24
  developing forms of, 89–92
  and the hands, 187–88
  intentional, 89–91, 92
  mind's-eye, 89–90, 92
  and psychometry, 187, 223–24, 238
  spontaneous, 89–90, 91–92
claustrophobia, 174–75
clearing and balancing, 3
color(s), 211–35
  affirmations for, 242
  attributes, 221–22
  of auras, 178, 183, 213, 218
  awareness of needs, 232–35
  of chakras, 159, 161–62
  and culture, 213–14
  in daily life, healing via, 224–27,
    237–40, 241–42
  emotive relationship with, 211–12
  enhancing/depleting, 233–34
  frequencies of, 216
  healing via, 9, 220–21, 232–35
  health issues reference chart,
    250–52, 254

intuitive languages of, 215–17
intuitive vs. physiological pro-
    cessing of, 222–23
journaling (exercise), 230–31
and light, 212, 217–20
in meditation, 215–16, 227,
    229–30
meditation/healing practice, 228,
    237–43
as a multisensory language,
    223–24
perspectives on, 230–32
reflections (exercise), 230, 232
and science, 212–13
and sound, 216–17, 224
spectrum of, 212–13
and trust, 243
consciousness, definition of, 81, 118
corona discharge, 181
coronas, human. *See* auras
cosmic eggs, 157
cosmic rays, 219
Cousins, Gabriel, 225
crosses of Thor, 157

D

daimon (Divine), 85
Daly, Ray, 158
dark matter, 72
delayed luminescence, 111
DeLuca, John, 158
depression, biochemistry of, 16
diagnosis and recognition, 2
dialing up/down. *See* chakra(s),
    openness of
dielectric radiation, 110

dimensional doorways, 157
disease, and cellular malfunction, 111
distance education program, 247
Divine rays, 181
Divine Science of the Soul, 13–14
divine water, 110
DNA vibration, 111
dowsing, 25–26
Dunne, Brenda, 79–80

E

earth energy, 113–29
    adding more, 124–26
    affirmations, 139
    benefits, 113, *114–15*, 116–17,
        122–23
    in daily life, 138–39
    electromagnetic fields, 113,
        116–17
    enhancing/weakening, 126–29
    feelings of, 118
    gravitational fields, 116
    grounding via, 47, *114–15*,
        118–19, 122–23
    healing via, 8, 105, 119
    health issues reference chart, 251,
        253, 255
    journaling (exercise), 123–24,
        128–29
    ley lines, 116
    and love, 117–18
    meditation, 117, 131–38, 170–73
    pathways of, 120–22
    perspectives on, 122–23
    reflections (exercise), 123–24,
        136–38
    and trust, 139

    visualizing, 124
    vs. life-force energy, 121
Einstein, Albert, 52, 76, 77, 78
élan vital (life force), 110
electric body of health, 190–91
electric corona, 181
electromagnetic body, 181
electromagnetic fields, 113, 116–17,
    155, 183–84, 190
electromagnetic radiation/energy, 190
electromagnetic signals, 27–28
electrons, antioxidants as, 39
elima (aura), 180
emotions
    and color, 211–12
    emotional addiction, 73
    love, 117–18, 147
    and neuropeptides, 153
    in the present, 82–83
    repressed anger, 83
empathy, 24
endocrine gland(s)
    adrenal, 143, *146*
    and chakras, 143–44, *146*, 152–53,
        183
    pineal, 91, 143, *146*, 187, 223
    pituitary, 73, 91, 143, *146*
    thymus, 143, *146*
    thyroid, 143, *146*
energy
    Divine, 158
    energy points, 157
    humans as made of, 36–37
    as information, 154
    merging with other people's, 189
    See also auras; earth energy; life-
        force energy
energy body, 181

enlightenment, 12
entanglement theory, 80
entrainment, 228
environmental factors affecting well-being, 28
etheric body/force/web, 180, 181
etheric organs, 157
evolution, human, 22
exercises. *See* journaling; meditation(s); reflections
experiments, overview of, 6

F

feet chakras
dialing up/down, 267
earth-energy meditation, 133–34
earth-energy pathways through, 120
grounding via, 40, *41*
harmony of, 277
health issues reference chart, 253, 255
location/functions of, 143, *145–46*, 149
Fetzer Institute, 23
Finsen, Niels, 223
first chakra
grounding via, 40, *41*, 53
life-force/earth-energy meditation, 134
life-force/earth-energy pathways through, 120–21
location/functions of, 143–44, *145–46*, 147
formative cause, 109
Freemasons, 141
frequencies, 108–9, 178, 183–84, 189
Fylfot, 157

G

Gaia, 47, 123
See also earth energy
gestallung (life force), 110
glands. *See* endocrine gland(s)
The Gods Must Be Crazy, 214
golden bowls, 180
golden web, 181
gonads, 143, *146*
gravity, grounding via, 44–45, *46*, 62–65, 69
grounding, 39–60
affirmations, 69–70
anchor points, 40, *41*, 42 (*See also* auras; chakra(s); meditation sanctuary)
of auras, 179
benefits, 8, 39
children's, 54–56
concepts, 43–44
in daily life, 47–49, 68
definition of, 42–43, 44
via the earth, 47
via earth energy, *114–15*, 118–19, 122–23
via feeling, 50, 54
via gravity, 44–45, *46*, 62–65, 69
health issues reference chart, 251–52, 254
journaling (exercise), 57–58, 59, 67–68
via life-force energy, *114–15*, 122–23
meditation practices, 61–70, 168–70
reflections (exercise), 56–57, 58–59

via sound, 49–50, 52–54
and spiritual intelligence, 43
strong vs. weak, 58–59
via visualization, 49, 50–52

H

Hall, Manly P., 153
halos, 180
See also auras
hand chakras
dialing up/down, 266
harmony of, 276
health issues reference chart, 253,
255
life-force/earth-energy meditation, 135
location/functions of, 143,
145–46, 148
harmony, being in/out of, 136–38,
163–64, 168, 196–97, 231,
268–77
healing
of auras, 205–7, 209–10
via Bio-Acoustics, 108–9
via color, 9, 220–21, 224–27,
232–35, 237–42
distance study, 33–36
via earth energy, 8, 105, 119
and intuition, 22–23
via life-force energy, 8, 105, 119
via light, 9, 111–12, 223
and love, 117–18
See also meditation(s)
health aura, 181
health issues reference chart, 9,
249–55

Health Medicine Institute (Lafayette,
Calif.), 23
heliotherapy, 112
Higbie, Barbara, 52–53
Hill Park Clinic (Petaluma, Calif.),
23
Hippocrates, 109
holophonic sound, 54
huaca (aura), 180
Hubble, Edwin, 213
Hunt, Valerie, 107–8, 183, 216
hypothalamus, 73–74, *75*, 81, 91

I

images. *See* visualization
imagination in meditation, 158
Indira Gandhi National Centre for
the Arts, 142
inner voice, 85
insomnia, 123
instinct, 22
Institute of HeartMath, 117–18
Institute of Noetic Sciences, 27, 34
intention, perception empowered by,
80–81
International Society for the Study
of Subtle Energies and
Energy Medicine, 27
intuition
accessing, methods for, 2–3
accuracy of, 35–36
assessment, 31–37
author's personal experiences,
11–19
definition/characterization of,
21–22

intuition (*continued*)
    exploration, 2–3
    and healing, 22–23
    and knowledge, 156
    language of, 5, 21, 161, 188
    research, 33–36
    sense of, 28–29
    successes of, 23
    trust of, 7, 70
    types, 24–26
    and wisdom, 26, 156
    See also awareness, intuitive;
        grounding
Intuition Medicine
    clairvoyance training in the pro-
        gram, 89–92
    in daily life, 7
    entrance requirements, 8
    overview, 3
intuitive awareness. *See* awareness,
    intuitive
intuitive body, 181

J

Jahn, Robert, 78, 79–80
Jainism, 142
James, William, 85
jaundice in newborns, 227
Jesuits, 141
journaling
    chakras, 163–64
    color, 230–31
    daily use, 246
    earth energy, 123–24, 128–29
    on grounding, 57–58, 59, 67–68
    life-force energy, 123–24, 128–29

    on meditation sanctuary, 92–96,
        102–3
    purposes, 4
Jung, Carl, 110

K

Kirlian auras, 181
Kirlian cameras, 27
Klotsche, Charles, 217
knowing/knowledge
    assessment, 32–33, 36
    characterization of, 25
    and intuition, 156
    perception empowered by, 80–81
    vs. wisdom, 52
Krishnamurti, J., 18
kundalini (a yogic life force), 12

L

labyrinths, 152, 157
Leonardo da Vinci, 212
ley lines, 116
L-Field, 181
life centers, 157
life-force energy
    adding more, 124–26
    affirmations, 139
    auras created by, 180–81
    benefits, 122–23
    body of light-force, 110–12
    in chakras, 155–56
    concepts comparable to, 109–10
    in daily life, 138–39
    definition of, 106
    enhancing/weakening, 126–29
    feelings of, 113

grounding via, *114–15*, 122–23
healing via, 8, 105, 119
health issues reference chart, 251,
    253, 255
journaling (exercise), 123–24,
    128–29
life as energy and medicine, 105–7
life-force vibration, 107–13
and light/vibration, 112–13
meditation, 131–32, 134–38,
    170–73
nadis, 106
pathways of, 120–22
perspectives on, 122–23
reflections (exercise), 123–24,
    136–38
and trust, 139
visualizing, 124
vs. earth energy, 121
light
    benefits, 112–13
    body of light-force, 110–12
    and color, 212, 217–20
    as energy, 217–18
    healing via, 9, 111–12, 223
    intensity of, 218
    and matter, 112
    normal vs. coherent, 106
    therapy using, 111–12, 223
    wavelengths of, 218–19
    wheels/circles of, 157
    white, 212
    See also auras
light body, 181
lines of the world, 180
liquor vitae (life force), 109
love, 117–18, 147
luminescence, delayed, 111

M

magnale magnum (life force), 110
magnetism, electricity, and light, 213
magnetoelectricity, 181
malillumination, 112
manilu (life force), 109
Mara, 50
Master of Intuition Medicine, 33
materialistic worldview, 156–57
matter, 119
McCluskey, Ann, 23
medical intuitives, 23
medicine, alternative vs. West-
    ern/traditional, 22–23, 162
    See also acupuncture
medieval alchemy, 110
meditation(s)
    analytical, 158
    audio recordings, 6, 246
    for auras, 194–95, 201–2, *203,*
        204–10, 237–40
    brain waves slowed by, 228
    and coherence in the brain, 106
    color in, 215–16, 227, 229–30
    color meditation, 228, 237–43
    contemplative, 100–102, 132–36,
        161–62, 167–68, 201–2,
        237–40
    earth-energy, 117, 131–38, 170–74,
        237–40
    for grounding, 61–70, 168–70,
        237–40
    grounding/meditation sanctu-
        ary/life-force/earth-
        energy/aura/chakra/color,
        237–40
    health practice of, 81–82

meditation(s) (*continued*)
  life-force energy, 131–32, 134–38,
    170–74, 237–40
  and living in the present, 8
  as a location, 8 (*See also* medita-
    tion sanctuary)
  mindfulness, 158
  overview, 5–6
  preparation, 6
  prone gravity-grounding, 62–65
  rainbow, 237–39
  seated grounding, 65–67
  timing of, 6
  visualization/imagination in, 158
  See also meditation sanctuary
meditation sanctuary, 8, 71–97, 75
  affirmations for, 87, 104
  being in the present, 82–84,
    93–94, 96
  color meditation, 237–40
  in daily life, 86, 103
  experiments, 103–4
  and the future, 78–79
  grounding via, 40, 41, 63
  health issues reference chart, 251,
    253, 255
  images for, 88–89
  and intuitive inquiry, 101–2
  journaling (exercise), 92–96,
    102–3
  light within, 82
  and the Now, 71–74, 76–77, 83–84
  perceiving your own reality,
    79–81
  and perception, 84–86
  practice, 99–104
  reflections (exercise), 92, 95, 97
  as a sacred place, 87–89

and trust, 104
and vision, 82, 84–86, 91
megbe (aura), 180
memories, painful, 73
Menninger Clinic, 27
mental body, 181
mind, past/future affected by, 78–79
mitogenetic radiation, 181
Mother Earth, 47, 113, 116
  See also earth energy
munia (aura), 180
music, 52–54
mystic mazes, 157
mystics, brain waves of, 113

N

nadis (energy networks), 106
Nakagawa, Kyoichi, 117
Namaste (Hindu greeting), 104
National Institute of Complementary and Alternative Medicine, 23
nefish (aura), 180
negative energy, 120–21
nerve plexuses, 157
neuropeptides, 152–53
Newton, Isaac, 212, 213, 216, 218
ngai (life force), 109
nimbuses, 180
9 Corners Center for Balanced
  Living (Novato, Calif.), 23
noetic (direct knowing), 85
noetic energy, 181
Now, 71–74, 76–77, 83–84
  See also present, being
N-rays, 180
nuos (aura), 180

O

odic force, 110
orgone, 110

P

pancreas, 143, *146*
Paracelsus, 109, 180
paraelectricity, 181
paramanu (aura), 180
PEAR (Princeton Engineering
    Anomalies Research) labora-
    tory, 27, 79–80
pentacles, 157
perception
    of auras, clairvoy-
        ant/clairaudient, 177–78,
        187
    and meditation sanctuary,
        84–86
    of time, 74, 76
    visualization/knowing/intention
        as empowering, 80–81
Pert, Candace, 73
photoreception in the skin, 223
photo-repair, 110–11
physics, 156
pineal gland, 91, 143, *146*, 187, 223
pituitary gland, 73, 91, 143, *146*
Plato, 52, 85, 180
pneuma (aura), 180
Popp, Fritz-Albert, 111, 187
portals, 157
prana (life force), 109
precognition, 25, 32–33
prephysical energy, 181
present, being, 82–84, 93–94, 96

See also Now
Princeton Engineering Anomalies
    Research (PEAR) laboratory,
        27, 79–80
protection/self-possession, 3
Psi faculty, 110
psi plasma, 181
psychokinesis, 78–79
psychometry
    assessment, 32–33, 36
    characterization of, 25–26
    and clairvoyance, 187, 223–24,
        238
    grounding via, 54
    to measure life-force energy,
        155–56
psychotechnics meters, 27
Pythagoras, 156

Q

quantum biology, 105
quantum mechanics/physics, 80, 110,
    213, 217

R

random number generators, 27
Receive Spirit, 19
reflections
    auras, 196–98
    chakras, 163–64
    colors, 230, 232
    earth energy, 123–24, 136–38
    grounding, 56–57, 58–59
    life-force energy, 123–24, 136–38
    meditation sanctuary, 92, 95, 97
relativity theory, 52, 76
Resonant Field Imaging™, 27

rlun (aura), 180
Rosicrucian roses, 157
Rosicrucians, 18, 141
ruach (aura), 180

S

sacred discs, 157
sacred gateways, 157
Samueli Institute, 23
Saputo, Len, 111
Schlitz, Marilyn, 78–79
Schmidt, Helmut, 78–79
Schumann Resonance, 113
science
    bioelectric fields measured by, 27
    and color, 212–13
    and spirituality, 156–57
sentics, 53–54
Sephiroths, 157
seven, symbolism of, 153
seven churches, 157
seven-circuit labyrinth, 157
seven lamps, 157
sila (aura), 180
Singapore Red Swastika Hospital,
    142
Singh, Sant Kirpal, 14
skin, 223
Society for Scientific Exploration, 27
Socrates, 85
solar crosses, 157
solar orbs, 180
sonic frequencies, 108–9
Sonnenrad, 157
sound
    and color, 216–17, 224
    grounding via, 49–50, 52–54

sonic frequencies, 108–9
Sound Wave Energy tapes, 53
space-time continuum, 77, 78
spiritual fire, 181
Spiritual Incarnation System™, 19
spirituality/spiritual intelligence
    in auras, 186
    body–spirit unity, 156–57
    definition of, 81
    and grounding, 43
    and science, 156–57
    spiritual skin, 181
*Spiritual Nutrition and the Rainbow
    Diet* (Cousins), 225
spiritus (life force), 110
stars, composition of, 213
Sufis, 52
superstring theory, 105–6
svasticas/swastikas, 157
synchronicity, 110
synergy, 110
synesthesia, 223–24, 238

T

telepathic chakras
    dialing up/down, 265
    harmony of, 275
    health issues reference chart, 253,
        255
    location/functions of, 143,
        145–46, 149
telepathy, 25, 32–33
telesma (aura), 180
Theosophists, 110, 141, 142
Theresa, Saint, 16
thousand-petalled lotuses, 157
thymus gland, 143, *146*

thyroid gland, 143, *146*
Tiller, William, 108, 181, 183
time, 74, 76–78
Tolle, Eckhart, 71–72
Transcendentist™ (Berkeley), 23
transpersonal psychology, 85
trees of life, 157
triskelion, 157
Truman, Harry, 157
trust
    and auras, 210
    and chakra, 176
    and color, 243
    and earth energy, 139
    and life-force energy, 139
    and meditation sanctuary, 104

U

universe, expansion of, 213

V

vibration, life-force, 107–13
victimhood, 73
vision, 82, 84–86, 91
    See also clairvoyance
vis medicatrix naturae (life force), 109
visualization
    of auras, 193–94
    of color, 215–16
    for earth energy, 124
    grounding through, 49, 50–52
    for life-force energy, 124
    in meditation, 158
    for meditation sanctuary, 88–89
    perception empowered by, 80–81
vital fluid, 110
Vitalists, 110
vitality sheath, 181
vivaxis, 47
voll meters, 27
vortices, 157

W

wakan (aura), 180
web of frequency/light, 181
What the Bleep Do We Know?! 73
wheels of light, 157
whirling wheel, 141–42
Whitman, Walt, 224
wisdom, 26, 52, 156
wisdom wheels, 159–60
wodan (aura), 180
worry, 154

X

X-Force, 110
X-rays, 219

Y

yesod (aura), 180

Z

Zajonc, Arthur, 82

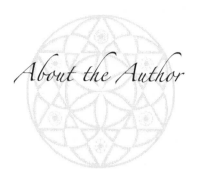

About the Author

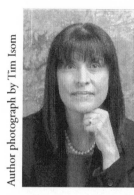

Author photograph by Tim Isom

*F*rancesca McCartney, PhD, is founder and president of the Academy of Intuition Medicine in Sausalito, California. The Academy offers a master's degree in Intuition Medicine and is a continuing education provider to CMT, LCSW, MFT practitioners, and registered nurses. Since 1984, Dr. McCartney has trained students to use her techniques in their work as health-care providers, physical therapists, and counselors. She has been practicing and developing her intuitive skills for thirty years and has a dual PhD in Intuition Medicine and Energy Medicine. Francesca frequently speaks to complementary and alternative medicine organizations and is widely published in professional journals on the topic of Intuition Medicine. She lives in Marin County, California.

For more information on the Academy of Intuition Medicine contact:
P.O. Box 1921, Mill Valley, California 94942
Phone: 415-381-1010 • Fax: 415-381-1080
www.IntuitionMedicine.org • Francesca@IntuitionMedicine.org